PTCB
EXAM PREP
2024-2025

PHARMACY TECHNICIAN MASTERY

The Ultimate Guide to Acing the PTCB Exam with
Proven Strategies, Q&A and Practice Tests

Vere Simonds

TABLE OF CONTENTS

INTRODUCTION

The decision to pursue PTCB certification is an invaluable step towards solidifying your commitment to professional excellence in pharmacy care. This book provides detailed insights, practical knowledge, and extensive practice material, ensuring all aspects of the Pharmacy Technician Certification Board (PTCB) Exam are thoroughly covered.

In these pages, you will discover why earning your certification is not just a rite of passage but an integral part of a fulfilling career in healthcare. As the role of pharmacy technicians evolves, the importance of having a robust understanding of pharmaceutical practices becomes increasingly critical. This introduction will elucidate the growing demands for competent pharmacy technicians and illustrate how passing the PTCB Exam elevates your professional status, enriches your career prospects, and empowers you to make a positive impact in patient care.

Each chapter of this book has been meticulously organized to mirror the subjects and format found within the actual PTCB Exam. Our goal is to familiarize you with everything from legal requirements and ethical standards to prescription management and medication safety—while also enhancing your problem-solving skills through practical calculations and real-world scenarios.

Why focus so intently on the PTCB Exam? Earning certification demonstrates your dedication and expertise, distinguishing you in a competitive field. It's tangible proof of your ability to uphold stringent pharmaceutical standards, thus affording patients peace of mind that their health is in well-trained hands. This certification can open doors to advanced roles within pharmacy operations and beyond.

As you delve into this preparatory material, remember that each topic covered serves as both a learning module and a stepping stone towards your goal. Remaining focused on the benefit of becoming certified will motivate you during your studies and help align your efforts with success.

Let *"PTCB Exam Prep"* be your champion in this endeavor—we're here to support you from the very first page until the moment you receive that pass notification. Turn this page and take that first bold step towards mastery and professional achievement.

CHAPTER 1
INTRODUCTION TO THE PTCB EXAM

Understanding the PTCB Certification

The Pharmacy Technician Certification Board (PTCB) sets a benchmark for pharmacy technicians that not only aims to validate their knowledge but also to enhance the quality of service in pharmaceutical care. So what does this certification involve, and why is it so crucial for those plying their trade in pharmacy tech?

The PTCB Certification is recognized across the United States and is often a mandatory stepping stone for technicians who aim to take their careers to the next level. It signifies a standard of excellence and a commitment to ethical practices and continuous learning within the pharmacy community.

One begins this path by meeting specific criteria. The candidate must have a high school diploma or GED equivalent, clean criminal record, and may be required to have completed an educational program or have equivalent work experience in a pharmacy setting. Once these preliminary requirements are met, the aspiring technician can apply for the Pharmacy Technician Certification Exam (PTCE).

The PTCE is composed of multiple-choice questions designed to assess a technician's knowledge across several domains critical to effective pharmacy practice. These include but are not limited to medications, federal laws and regulations, patient safety protocols, medication order entry and fill process, inventory management, billing, reimbursement procedures, and information systems. Each domain reflects real-life scenarios that a certified pharmacy technician would encounter.

Successful completion of the PTCE culminates in obtaining the Certified Pharmacy Technician (CPhT) credential. This certification is valid for two years after which the technician must complete continuing education (CE) credits to maintain their certified status. This requirement underscores the importance of remaining current with evolving practices and standards in an industry where patient health and well-being are at stake.

Beyond merely passing an exam, PTCB certified technicians demonstrate higher aptitude in various aspects of their job role. They tend to have better job prospects with higher earning potential compared to non-certified counterparts. Certification can also serve as a springboard towards further specialization within pharmacy tech roles such as compounding or chemotherapy mixing thereby elevating professional practice standards.

The importance of the PTCB Certification cannot be understated in terms of patient safety. Certified technicians form an integral cog in healthcare, ensuring that medications are dispensed accurately and responsibly. In doing so, they uphold public health objectives by minimizing medication errors which can have serious implications.

Moreover, PTCB Certification promotes professional solidarity among pharmacy technicians. There emerges an inherent community striving towards excellence where knowledge sharing becomes commonplace leading to enhanced cohesiveness in pharmacy operations.

Given these facets, it's evident why delving into the world of PTCB Certification requires dedication and commitment. Not only do you need to understand drugs and their effects but you also need to navigate regulations and execute procedures meticulously within various health care environments.

As part of your preparation for this pivotal pathway, embrace structured study plans inclusive of both theory fundamentals and practical examples that mirror real-world applications. Consider joining study groups or online forums where collective wisdom can be tapped into enriching your knowledge base beyond textbook material.

Invest in quality study materials; look for books or online resources that come recommended by professionals who have successfully trodden this path before you. These preparative steps are crucial aiming towards not just passing the PTCE but excelling at it paving your trajectory as a distinguished member within the echelons of pharmacy technicians.

Importance of Becoming a Certified Pharmacy Technician

Pharmacy technicians are an integral part of the healthcare team, playing a key role in managing the complexities of medication distribution and patient care. While on-the-job experience is valuable, becoming a certified pharmacy technician (CPhT) through the Pharmacy Technician Certification Board (PTCB) demonstrates a higher level of commitment and proficiency.

Certification serves as a benchmark of excellence and is often a requirement for employment in many health systems and pharmacies. By becoming certified, pharmacy technicians not only prove their skills but also signal to employers that they are serious about their profession. Here are several reasons why acquiring a PTCB certification is essential.

Certification ensures standardized knowledge and skills. The PTCB's ExCPT exam covers critical areas such as pharmacology, pharmacy law and regulations, medication safety, and quality assurance — all of which are necessary to practice safely and effectively. This rigorous exam prepares candidates for real-world scenarios that they will encounter in their day-to-day duties.

Certified pharmacy technicians often have a competitive advantage in the job market. Employers prefer hiring individuals who have gone the extra mile to validate their competence through certification, as this reflects a sincere dedication to their professional development. In many cases, holding a PTCB certification can lead to better job opportunities including positions with greater responsibility and oversight.

Furthermore, being a certified pharmacy technician could lead to higher earnings. Many employers offer increased pay rates for technicians who hold certifications because they bring recognized skills and knowledge that contribute to more efficient operations. Salaries can vary widely based on location, experience, and other factors; however, certification consistently correlates with higher income.

Certification also opens doors to career advancement. For ambitious technicians eager to progress within their careers, certification is often the first step towards positions like pharmacy manager or even transitioning into roles such as pharmaceutical sales representatives or health information technicians.

Patient safety is another crucial aspect of pharmaceutical care where certified technicians make an impact. By demonstrating mastery of medication management principles and practices through certification, these professionals help minimize errors in medication dispensing — a vital task considering the potentially grave consequences of mistakes in this area.

Moreover, maintaining certification requires ongoing education. This requirement ensures that pharmacy technicians stay current with latest best practices and evolving regulations within an ever-changing healthcare landscape. The commitment to continuous improvement is not only beneficial for individual growth but also improves the healthcare system as a whole by guaranteeing knowledgeable staff.

The peer recognition that comes with being certified cannot be underestimated either. Achieving this professional milestone boosts both personal pride and reputation among colleagues within the industry. This recognition solidifies one's status as an expert among peers which can inspire respect and open up further networking opportunities within the field.

Achieving PTCB certification generates numerous benefits for pharmacy technicians seeking to enhance their credentials and advance their careers within health care services. Not only does it equip these professionals with necessary knowledge and skills required to excel but also provides external validation of their expertise — making it evident why this achievement holds such significance in today's market.

By taking into account all these factors along with continuing technological advancements affecting drug therapy management and pharmacy operations overall– it becomes clear: the PTCB certification is more than just a set of initials behind one's name; it's an essential investment in one's future within the healthcare industry. Aspiring pharmacy technicians should consider this crucial step towards personal development not merely as an option but as an imperative move for anyone serious about thriving professionally within this sector.

Overview of the PTCB Exam Structure

The PTCB exam is designed to evaluate the knowledge and skills necessary to work as a pharmacy technician and ensure that certified individuals meet the National Healthcare Association's standards. The PTCB exam is a computer-based test (CBT) composed of 90 multiple-choice questions. Among these, 80 questions are scored, and the remaining 10 are not scored but rather used to gather statistical data to inform future exam questions. These 10 unscored questions are indistinguishable from the scored ones, so candidates should treat each question with equal importance.

The examination is divided into four major categories, each category focusing on a crucial aspect of pharmacy technology practice. These domains reflect the actual duties of a pharmacy technician and are updated periodically to reflect changes in practice and regulations. The four primary knowledge domains are:

To ensure fairness and comprehensive coverage of all relevant topics, the questions on the PTCB exam are divided into four knowledge domains, each reflecting key areas of understanding required by pharmacy technicians:

1. **Medications:** This domain tests your familiarity with different types of medications, their generic and brand names, classifications, side effects, and therapeutic purposes. It also assesses your knowledge of standard dosages and necessary precautions or contraindications when handling medication. Approximately 40% of the exam will cover content from this domain.

2. **Federal Requirements:** Being a competent pharmacy technician also involves a thorough understanding of the legal aspects governing pharmacy practice. This section includes questions about regulatory standards, record-keeping requirements, controlled substance laws, and quality assurance principles. It constitutes roughly 12.5% of the total examination.

3. **Patient Safety and Quality Assurance:** Patient care is paramount in healthcare settings; therefore, approximately 26.25% of the PTCB exam focuses on practices that ensure patient safety and promote quality services in pharmacies. You'll find questions about prescription order processing procedures, error prevention strategies, as well as safety measures in medication dispensation.

4. **Order Entry and Processing:** The remaining portion of the exam - approximately 21.25%, centers on evaluating your ability to process medication orders accurately. This encompasses interpretation of prescriptions, calculation skills needed for preparation and dispensation of drugs, inventory management techniques, billing processes, and reimbursement procedures.

Candidates are allotted two hours to finish the PTCB exam. Efficient time management during the test allows examinees time to carefully consider each question without rushing through sections towards the end of their allotted time.

Preparing for the PTCB exam requires comprehensive study across all domains. While various study materials are available—ranging from textbooks specifically designed for PTCB preparation to online courses and practice exams—the best preparation comes from hands-on experience gained through working in a pharmacy setting under a qualified pharmacist's supervision.

As scoring goes for the PTCB exam, it uses a scaled score system ranging from 1000 to 1600 points. To pass the examination successfully, a candidate needs to achieve a score of at least 1400 points—an indicator that they possess sufficient knowledge and skill level required for certification.

Upon completion of the exam at an authorized testing center, preliminary results are available immediately; however official results and certification notifications typically arrive within three weeks post-exam via mail or email, depending on state laws and candidate preferences.

Understanding how scores are calculated is crucial as well since it can inform candidates about areas requiring further study should they need to retake the exam due to an unsuccessful attempt. A detailed score report highlights performance in each subject area—thereby providing valuable feedback about knowledge gaps to address.

CHAPTER 2

THE ROLE OF A PHARMACY TECHNICIAN

Responsibilities and Duties

The role of a pharmacy technician not only significantly affects the operations within a pharmacy but also influences patient care and safety. It is important to recognize the interaction between a technician's competency and the overall efficiency of pharmaceutical services. As gatekeepers of medication distribution, their precision, knowledge, and ethical standards directly impact patients' health outcomes. A pharmacy technician's role encompasses various duties that facilitate pharmacists' work and ensure a smooth workflow within pharmacies.

1. **Medication Preparation and Dispensing:** One of your primary responsibilities will be preparing and dispensing medications to patients. This includes counting tablets, measuring amounts of medication for prescriptions, compounding or mixing medications, and packaging and labeling prescriptions. You might also prepare intravenous (IV) mixtures under a pharmacist's supervision in hospital settings.

2. **Controlled Substance Management:** Handling controlled substances requires utmost diligence. You will maintain inventories, track controlled substance transactions, and work closely with pharmacists to ensure compliance with all regulatory requirements. Accurate record-keeping is key in this area to avoid potential legal issues.

3. **Patient Interaction and Support:** Pharmacy technicians often serve as the first point of contact for patients. You'll be responsible for collecting patient information necessary for processing prescriptions—this includes verifying insurance details and obtaining

authorizations when required. Enterprising technicians may take an extra step by participating in patient education regarding medication use, storage, and side effects under pharmacist guidance.

4. **Order Entry and Processing:** Prescription processing involves entering prescription and insurance information into the computer system and ensuring that the correct medication is provided in the right quantity and dosage form. Here lies an important duty—accurate data entry prevents potential medication errors.

5. **Inventory Management:** Monitoring inventory is essential for any pharmacy's operation. Your role will involve stocking shelves, rotating stock to ensure the use of older medications first, ordering supplies when necessary, keeping records up-to-date for reordering purposes, and removing expired or damaged drugs from inventory.

6. **Insurance Claim Handling:** Competency with insurance claims handling can significantly improve patient satisfaction as well as pharmacy efficiency. You'll be dealing with third-party insurance billing; including reconciling claims, addressing rejects or denials, ensuring proper billing practices are followed, while simultaneously liaising with insurance providers to resolve issues swiftly.

7. **Compliance With Regulations:** A substantial part of your duties extends into ensuring that all activities comply with state laws and regulations pertaining to pharmacy practice. These regulations concern patient confidentiality (HIPAA), safe handling procedures (OSHA), quality assurance protocols, and more.

8. **Equipment Operation:** In various settings, technicians are also required to operate machinery like tablet counters, mixers or compounders, label printers etc., keeping them clean and functioning properly. You should always follow safety guidelines while operating such equipment to prevent accidents or contamination.

9. **Continued Education:** To keep up with advances in pharmaceuticals pharmacists require ongoing education—a responsibility extending to technicians as well. State boards often mandate specific continuing education credits for technician certification renewal—sustaining your competency within an evolving field.

These responsibilities form the pillars upon which pharmacy technicians build their careers—a balance between technical proficiency, attention to detail, interpersonal skills, commitment to patient safety—and above all—a strong ethical foundation that guides you through your day-to-day tasks within any pharmacy setting.

Pharmacy Technician Code of Ethics

The Code of Ethics provides the bedrock for professional conduct and decision-making. Adherence to these ethical standards guarantees that patients receive optimal care, their privacy is respected, and that decisions made are free from bias or misconduct. The

Pharmacy Technician Code of Ethics acts as a guiding light that illuminates the path of professionalism, respect, and accountability, which are indispensable elements in fostering a trustworthy healthcare system.

The Code of Ethics consists of several key principles that ensure patient welfare, uphold the integrity of the profession, and foster collaboration within healthcare.

1. **Commitment to Patient Health and Safety:** The foremost priority for pharmacy technicians is the health and safety of patients. Technicians are obligated to maintain and improve their professional competencies, stay informed about new medications and technologies, and adhere strictly to established procedures for dispensing medications. They must always ensure the right patient receives the right medication, in the correct dosage, and with clear instructions, thus minimizing medication errors.

2. **Upholding Professional Competence:** Pharmacy technicians must acknowledge the limitations of their knowledge and skills and only undertake tasks for which they are appropriately trained and authorized. Continuing education is vital; technicians must seek ongoing opportunities to learn and grow within their field while adhering to legal requirements and ethical standards.

3. **Respect for Confidentiality:** Confidentiality is paramount in maintaining trust with patients. Pharmacy technicians are privy to sensitive personal health information and must protect it diligently. This involves complying with all relevant legislation related to privacy rights and ensuring that any information is accessed only by authorized individuals as necessary for patient care.

4. **Integrity in Relationships:** A pharmacy technician's relationships with colleagues, other healthcare professionals, patients, and society at large should be marked by honesty and integrity. This means communicating clearly, avoiding conflicts of interest, not engaging in fraudulent activities or deceitful practices, and being accountable for one's actions.

5. **Supporting Colleagues in Their Professional Development:** Sharing knowledge with fellow pharmacy technicians supports a collective increase in professional standards. Contributing to discussions, mentoring newcomers to the profession, and participating in professional organizations are some ways pharmacy technicians can actively engage in uplifting their colleagues.

6. **Professional Behavior:** Pharmacy technicians should conduct themselves with professionalism at all times. This includes dressing appropriately for a healthcare setting, using respectful language with patients and co-workers regardless of stress levels or provocation, managing time efficiently, showing resilience under pressure, striving for excellence in every task performed.

7. **Advocacy for Quality Improvement:** Being actively involved in efforts that aim to improve medication safety practices reflects a deep commitment to patient care.

Pharmacy technicians should be advocates both within their place of employment – suggesting improvements where necessary – and also within the wider community by educating others about safe medication practices.

8. **Compliance with Laws and Regulations:** Beyond ethical considerations is the legal specter that regulates pharmacy practice. Technicians must comply with all federal, state/provincial/territorial laws regulations that affect pharmacy services including those related to prescription drugs control substances administration.

Ethics goes beyond mere compliance; however—it is about doing right even when not being watched or regulated. The true mark of an ethical pharmacy technician lies not just in adherence to rules but also in an innate understanding respect for human dignity.

Interactions with pharmacists and patients are a pivotal part of healthcare that ensures the effective delivery of medication therapy and patient care. An understanding of this dynamic is crucial for pharmacy technicians preparing for the Pharmacy Technician Certification Board (PTCB) exam.

Interactions with Pharmacists and Patients

Effective communication between pharmacists and patients is the foundation upon which successful health outcomes are built. The role of a pharmacist involve the verification of prescriptions, identification of drug interactions, and providing medication counseling. When patients visit pharmacies, they expect not only to receive their medications but also to obtain information that will help them use their medications safely and effectively.

1. **Clear Communication:** Clear communication is at the heart of every pharmacist-patient interaction. As a pharmacy technician, you must be able to convey information accurately and ask pertinent questions to ensure patients understand their treatment regimens. This includes explaining dosage instructions, potential side effects, and how to store medications properly.

2. **Empathy and Trust:** Empathy plays an essential role in building trust with patients. By demonstrating understanding and compassion towards a patient's needs and concerns, you create a comfortable environment for them to discuss sensitive health issues. This trust encourages patients to be open about their medication experiences, leading to better personalized care.

3. **Confidentiality:** Confidentiality is crucial in any healthcare setting. Patients need to feel confident that their personal health information is protected. As a pharmacy technician, handle sensitive data with discretion and ensure that privacy laws are always adhered to.

4. **Cultural Competence:** Pharmacists and pharmacy technicians should be culturally competent, recognizing the diverse backgrounds of the patients they serve.

Understanding cultural influences on health beliefs and practices ensures that all advice and education given are respectful to the individual's values and perspectives.

5. **Educating Patients:** The education of patients about their medications contributes significantly to adherence rates. Topics such as the importance of completing a course of antibiotics or managing chronic conditions like diabetes are often addressed by pharmacists but supported by technicians who reinforce these messages through pamphlets or answering follow-up questions.

6. **Overcoming Barriers:** Barriers such as language differences or health literacy issues can impede communication. Pharmacy professionals should be prepared to address these challenges through tools like translation services or easy-to-understand visual aids that simplify complex information.

7. **Handling Complaints:** Dealing with patient complaints can be challenging but it provides an opportunity for quality improvement within the pharmacy setting. Effective complaint resolution involves active listening, acknowledging the issue without assigning blame, finding a resolution or compromise, and following up on customer satisfaction.

8. **Medication Safety:** A significant aspect of pharmacist-patient interaction involves ensuring medication safety by preventing errors, checking for allergies, drug interactions, contraindications, and advising on safe administration practices.

9. **Collaboration With Healthcare Professionals:** Pharmacists frequently collaborate with other healthcare professionals to provide integrated care for patients. As part of this team-based approach, pharmacy technicians support coordination efforts by managing communications between pharmacists and prescribing physicians or other healthcare providers.

10. **Workflow Efficiency:** In order for pharmacists to interact meaningfully with patients, efficient workflow practices must be maintained within the pharmacy. Technicians contribute by managing inventory effectively, processing prescriptions expediently, triaging concerns that may need pharmacist intervention thereby maximizing the time pharmacists have available for direct patient care.

11. **Professional Development:** Continuous professional development helps pharmacy technicians stay informed about new medications, treatment guidelines, technology advancements in dispensing medication etc., enabling them to better support both pharmacists in their clinical roles and patients in their journey towards wellness.

CHAPTER 3
PHARMACY LAW AND REGULATIONS

Federal and State Pharmacy Laws

Federal regulations ensure the safety and efficacy of drug distribution across the nation. The cornerstone of these regulations is the Food, Drug, and Cosmetic Act (FDCA) which empowers the U.S. Food and Drug Administration (FDA) to oversee drug approval, drug labeling, and pharmaceutical advertising. Under the FDCA, medications are classified into prescription and over-the-counter drugs, with distinct rules governing each category.

Another significant legislation is the Controlled Substances Act (CSA), which categorizes all substances that have potential for abuse into five schedules based on their likelihood for dependency, with Schedule I representing drugs with no accepted medical use and a high potential for abuse such as heroin, and Schedule V including substances that have lower potential for abuse such as cough preparations containing a small amount of codeine. The Drug Enforcement Administration (DEA) enforces compliance with the CSA, and every pharmacy must register with the DEA to dispense controlled substances.

The Combat Methamphetamine Epidemic Act (CMEA) also demands attention as it sets daily and monthly limits on over-the-counter sales of pseudoephedrine and ephedrine products used in manufacturing methamphetamine. Records of sales in logbooks are required for transactions exceeding specified limits.

State laws and regulations expand upon federal mandates, focusing more directly on pharmacy practice standards within state boundaries. Though each state has its own set of laws, there are commonalities among them. State Boards of Pharmacy regulate licensure requirements for pharmacists and pharmacy technicians, oversee practice standards in both community and institutional settings, ensure compliance with continuing education requirements, manage drug dispensing protocols, and enforce disciplinary actions when necessary.

One key area where states exercise their authority is in defining technician roles and duties. Tasks such as medication dispensing can only be performed under direct supervision of licensed pharmacists, while in some states technicians may be authorized to perform additional duties including vaccine administration or checking technician-prepared medications under certain circumstances.

In adherence to state regulations on controlled substances, pharmacies are often required to use Prescription Drug Monitoring Programs (PDMPs), databases that track prescribing and dispensing schedules II-V controlled substances to prevent substance abuse. Through PDMPs, pharmacists can identify patients who may be doctor shopping or at risk of addiction.

States also mediate collaborative practice agreements (CPAs) between pharmacists and other healthcare providers. These CPAs detail how pharmacists can provide patient care services within their scope of practice which includes modifying medication therapy under predetermined protocols.

It is imperative for pharmacy technicians to remain vigilant about sterile compounding practices too. Following the tragic fungal meningitis outbreak linked to compounded sterile products in 2012, states have been tightening regulations to adhere closely to USP Chapter <797> guidelines on sterile compounding.

Likewise important are laws regarding patient privacy which align with federal Health Insurance Portability and Accountability Act (HIPAA). Both federal statutes and state laws impose stringent rules against unauthorized disclosure of patient health information.

Lastly, an understanding of generic substitution laws is essential. While federal law allows generic substitutions if deemed therapeutically equivalent by the FDA's Orange Book, it's state laws that often dictate when it is appropriate or mandatory to substitute a prescribed drug with a generic alternative unless otherwise specified by prescriber or patient preference.

For PTCB Exam candidates it's vital not only to learn the content but also understand practical application of these laws within day-to-day pharmacy operations. Realistic scenarios involving law-related questions could be part of your examination as they test not just knowledge but judgement. Remaining up-to-date with changes in law is equally important since pharmacy is an ever-evolving field where legislation continually adapts to new medical discoveries and societal demands.

Controlled Substances Regulations

Controlled substances are drugs that have a high potential for abuse and dependence, classified into schedules by the Drug Enforcement Administration (DEA) based on their medical use, potential for abuse, and safety or dependence liability.

The Controlled Substances Act (CSA) is the statute prescribing federal U.S. drug policy under which the manufacture, importation, possession, use, and distribution of certain substances are regulated. The Act lists substances into one of five schedules. Schedule I substances have a high potential for abuse, no currently accepted medical use in treatment in the United States, and a lack of accepted safety for use under medical supervision. Examples include heroin and LSD. Schedules II through V decrease in potential for abuse, with Schedule II drugs still having a high potential but with accepted medical uses. These include medications like oxycodone and fentanyl. Schedules III to V include substances like anabolic steroids and some antidiarrheals.

Pharmacy technicians must be adept at recognizing these classes of drugs due to the legal implications surrounding their handling. The DEA requires strict record keeping and inventory management for all schedules, but especially schedules II through V. A pharmacy must maintain accurate inventories and records of controlled substances transactions which are subject to inspection by the DEA.

In handling controlled substances prescriptions, technicians should be aware that Schedule II prescriptions require a written prescription from a licensed practitioner. However, under certain circumstances such as emergencies or when electronic prescribing is set up within the practitioner's practice as per DEA regulations, verbal orders may be acceptable.

Prescriptions for Schedule III-V drugs can be written or verbal and can be refilled up to five times within six months from the date of prescription if authorized by the prescriber. For Schedule II drugs, no refills are allowed; a new prescription must be written each time.

Another key point is regarding security measures within pharmacies. Controlled substances must be stored in a securely locked, substantially constructed cabinet or dispersed throughout the pharmacy's stock in such a manner as to obstruct thefts or diversion of large quantities.

The PTCB exam expects pharmacy technicians to also understand federal requirements versus state law when it comes to controlled substances regulations as states may enact laws that are more stringent than federal regulations but not less restrictive. Technicians must always adhere to both sets of laws but comply with the stricter law when there's a conflict.

Moreover, understanding DEA Form 222—a form required when ordering Schedule I and II controlled substances—and maintaining proper documentation is crucial. Likewise, when a controlled substance is deemed unfit for sale (expired or damaged), it must be placed in an area designated for outdated medications until disposed of according to DEA guidelines using DEA Form 41.

Pharmacy technicians need to know about specific documentation pertaining to dispensed controlled substances which includes details like patients' name and address, drug name, dosage form, strength, quantity dispensed, date dispensed, prescribing physician's name and DEA registration number along with the pharmacist's name who filled or checked out the prescription.

In addition to dispensing responsibilities associated with controlled substances regulations, pharmacy technicians must remain aware of drug diversion tactics that could impact the pharmacy's operation such as fraudulent prescriptions or theft by individuals including employees.

Lastly, an evolving aspect which technicians studying for PTCB exams should note is electronic prescribing of controlled substances (EPCS), which was implemented to reduce prescription forgery and ensure secure electronic record-keeping. Understanding these systems' workings is increasingly important as technology becomes more integrated into health care practices.

HIPAA and Patient Privacy

The term "HIPAA" refers to the Health Insurance Portability and Accountability Act that was enacted by the U.S. Congress in 1996. HIPAA has several goals, including streamlining the healthcare industry's inefficient administrative processes, ensuring the portability of health insurance coverage, and significantly - advocating for patient privacy.

Privacy of health information is not only a concern for patients but is also legally mandated. With the advancement of technology and digital record-keeping, concerns about privacy breaches have magnified. HIPAA addresses this by establishing national standards for electronic health care transactions and national identifiers for providers, health insurance plans, and employers. It also delineates the rights of individuals to their health information while setting boundaries on the use and disclosure of their health records.

HIPAA includes the Privacy Rule and the Security Rule, which are directly relevant to pharmacy technicians and other healthcare professionals. The Privacy Rule sets standards for when protected health information (PHI) may be used or disclosed. Patient consent is generally required for routine disclosures for treatment, payment, or healthcare operations but there are exceptions for certain public responsibilities such as public health reporting.

For instance, a pharmacy technician may process prescription refills, where PHI would be required to perform their job function effectively. In doing so, HIPAA mandates that the pharmacy tech must ensure the minimum necessary information is utilized to diminish unnecessary exposure of a patient's PHI.

Moreover, the Privacy Rule grants patients various rights regarding their own health information like obtaining a copy of their records or requesting corrections. These rights are substantial in empowering patients and fostering transparency within healthcare establishments.

Moving on to the Security Rule, it complements the Privacy Rule by laying down standards concerning electronic PHI (ePHI). Pharmacy technicians utilizing computer systems to manage patient data must understand that these systems need to be compliant with the security measures elucidated in HIPAA. This involves ensuring confidentiality, integrity, and availability through administrative, physical, and technical safeguards.

For example, technicians could engage in securing workstations and devices from unauthorized access or employing encryption when sending ePHI across open networks. Failing to adhere to these security protocols could lead to serious ramifications—both on an individual level with fines or job loss and at an organizational level with reputational harm or legal penalties.

HIPAA has stringent provisions regarding education and training that stipulate all individuals dealing with PHI or ePHI - including pharmacy technicians - should receive ongoing training on handling patient data appropriately. This ensures they remain abreast of any changes in legislation or best practices within their operational scope.

Nevertheless, despite these comprehensive rules and regulations set by HIPAA—breaches can occur; typically through lost devices containing ePHI, unauthorized access/disclosure by employees or cyber-attacks such as hacking/phishing schemes targeting healthcare systems. When a breach happens, HIPAA requires covered entities notify affected patients without undue delay—and no later than 60 days following the discovery of a breach.

Studying HIPAA compliance helps future pharmacy technicians appreciate the responsibilities that come with handling sensitive patient information—it provides benchmarks against which they can measure their own practices ensuring patients' rights are maintained while fulfilling legal requirements. Furthermore, this knowledge signifies professionalism in healthcare delivery—an aspect highly valued within any medical field discipline.

CHAPTER 4

PHARMACEUTICAL CALCULATIONS

Dosage Calculations

The cornerstone of pharmaceutical practice is the accurate calculation of medication dosages. Proper dosage ensures efficacy and avoids potentially dangerous medication errors. The PTCB exam will test your ability to accurately calculate dosages, which is a critical skill for any pharmacy technician.

When calculating dosages, there are several important units of measurement that you must be familiar with. Common units used in pharmacy include milligrams (mg), grams (g), liters (L), milliliters (mL), and units for insulin measurements. To begin, it is crucial to understand how to convert between these units, as medications can be prescribed in one unit and supplied in another.

Let's start with some basic conversions:

- 1 gram = 1000 milligrams
- 1 liter = 1000 milliliters
- Units are a measure of effect specific for certain drugs like insulin, not mass

The first step in dosage calculation is to carefully read the prescription or medication order. You'll need to determine the amount of drug prescribed and the way in which the medication is supplied. For example, if a patient is prescribed 250 mg of a medication and it's supplied as 500 mg per tablet, they would need half a tablet per dose.

Next, consider any specific patient factors that might impact dosage calculations such as age, weight, and renal function. Pediatric and geriatric patients often require special dosage considerations because their bodies process medications differently. Additionally, medications that are dosed based on weight require careful attention; this is often denoted as mg/kg (milligram per kilogram).

Mathematically speaking, there are several formulae that every pharmacy technician should know:

1. **To find the required number of units or tablets:** Required Dose / Supplied Dose = Number of Units or Tablets
2. **Weight-based dosages:** Required Dose (mg/kg) * Patient's Weight (kg) = Total Daily Dose
3. **IV flow rates:** Volume (mL) / Time (hr) = IV Flow Rate (mL/hr)

Let's put this knowledge into practice with an example question similar to what you might find on the PTCB exam:

Dr. Smith prescribes Amoxicillin 250 mg p.o. every 8 hours for a patient who weighs 45 kg. The drug comes in suspension form with a concentration of 200 mg/5mL.

First, determine how many mLs of Amoxicillin this patient would need per dose using our first formula:

> *Required Dose = Prescribed Dose*
> *Supplied Dose = Concentration per mL*

Calculating this leads to:

> *Required Dose (250 mg) / Supplied Dose (200 mg/5 mL)*
> *= 250 mg / ((200 mg / 5 mL))*
> *= (250 * 5) / 200*
> *= 1250 / 200*
> *= 6.25 mL*

So, the patient needs to take 6.25 mL every 8 hours.

Furthermore, complications may also arise when calculating doses for continuous intravenous infusions or when titrating doses up or down according to therapeutic drug monitoring.

When studying for your PTCB Exam, it's imperative that you practice these types of calculations extensively since accuracy is paramount in pharmacy practice. Mistakes in dosing can have significant consequences for patient care – it's more than just getting an answer correct on your pharmacy technician exam.

Tools available including pill cutters, graduated cylinders, and dosing calculators can be helpful aids but understanding the underlying principles will allow you to check that technology-produced results are reasonable.

Tips for mastering dosage calculations:

1. Practice converting between different units regularly.
2. Familiarize yourself with commonly used formulas.
3. Practice with actual prescription orders.
4. Use study groups or apps designed to simulate PTCB exam questions.
5. Always double-check your calculations.

Completing a chapter on 'Dosage Calculations' without exceeding practical examples illustrates that while understanding theory is necessary, application through various types of problems solidifies one's skill set – a strategy crucial for passing the PTCB exam and excelling as a proficient pharmacy technician.

IV Flow Rate Calculations

As a pharmacy technician studying for the PTCB exam, understanding how to calculate IV flow rates is an essential skill that ensures patient safety and medication efficacy. Calculating the IV flow rate involves determining the volume of fluid that should be infused into a patient over a specified period. This is typically measured in milliliters per hour (mL/hr). The formula for calculating the IV flow rate is:

IV Flow Rate (mL/hr) = Total Volume to be Infused (mL) / Infusion Time (hr)

To ensure precision, one must also consider factors such as drop factor, which is the number of drops per milliliter (gtt/mL), based on the specific IV set being used. The formula then expands to include this factor:

Drop Rate (gtt/min) = [Total Volume to be Infused (mL) ×
Drop Factor (gtt/mL)] / Total Infusion Time (min)

Now let's delve into specific examples to illustrate how these calculations are put into practice.

Example 1:

A physician orders 1000 mL of saline to be infused over 8 hours using an IV set with a drop factor of 15 gtt/mL. To find out the flow rate in mL/hr, divide the total volume by time:

IV Flow Rate = 1000 mL / 8 hr
IV Flow Rate = 125 mL/hr

Next, to determine the drop rate per minute:

Drop Rate = [1000 mL × 15 gtt/mL] / (8 hr × 60 min/hr)
Drop Rate = [15000 gtt] / 480 min
Drop Rate ≈ 31 gtt/min

Example 2:

The order is for a medication infusion of 500 mL to be delivered over a span of 12 hours using tubing with a drop factor of 20 gtt/mL.

IV Flow Rate = 500 mL / 12 hr
IV Flow Rate ≈ 41.67 mL/hr

For the drop rate:

Drop Rate = [500 mL × 20 gtt/mL] / (12 hr × 60 min/hr)
Drop Rate = [10000 gtt] / 720 min
Drop Rate ≈ 13.89 gtt/min

When setting up an IV infusion, it's vital also to understand how to adjust the flow rate if needed during patient care. If you notice that your patient's IV infusion is ahead or behind schedule—perhaps due to changes in patient condition or alterations in physician orders—you will need to recalculate and adjust the flow rate accordingly.

For instance, if halfway through infusing the first example above you find that only 400 mL has been infused rather than the expected 500 mL, you will need to increase the flow rate to ensure the remaining fluid is infused within the remaining time.

New IV Flow Rate for Remaining Volume:

Remaining Volume = Total Volume - Volume Already Infused
Remaining Volume = 1000 mL - 400 mL
Remaining Volume = 600 mL

Remaining Time = Total Time - Time Elapsed
Remaining Time = 8 hr - 4 hr
Remaining Time = 4 hr

New IV Flow Rate = Remaining Volume / Remaining Time
New IV Flow Rate = 600 mL / 4 hr
New IV Flow Rate = 150 mL/hr

As precision in these calculations can quite literally mean life or death, pharmacy technicians must be meticulous and practiced in their IV flow rate calculation skills. It's also paramount that technicians are familiar with different types of infusion pumps and gravity drip methods since these devices may require additional considerations.

Remembering these key points will not only help you succeed on your PTCB exam but will also ensure excellence in patient care. Practice with multiple questions involving various scenarios, focusing on accuracy and speed, as this will serve you well during both your examination and your career as a pharmacy technician.

Medication Conversions

Conversions between metric, apothecary, and household systems may be necessary in a pharmacy setting. The metric system is the most commonly used system in medicine due to its simplicity and worldwide acceptance. It consists primarily of units like grams (g) for weight, liters (L) for volume, and meters (m) for length.

One of the most frequent conversions you'll encounter is between milligrams (mg) and grams (g). It's crucial to remember that 1 g equals 1,000 mg. Similarly, converting micrograms (mcg) to milligrams involves knowing that 1 mg is equal to 1,000 mcg.

In liquid medications, converting milliliters (mL) to liters is often necessary. With 1 L equaling 1,000 mL, precision in conversion ensures correct dosage measurements. Moreover, interpreting orders in drops might require knowledge of the fact that there are approximately 20 drops in 1 mL when using a standard dropper.

Occasionally, the apothecary system might still be utilized, especially in prescriptions from certain providers or on labels of older medicines. Key units include grains (gr), drams (dr), ounces (oz), and pints (pt). One grain is roughly equivalent to 65 mg; therefore converting grains to milligrams or vice versa is necessary to administer the medication correctly as ordered.

Household measurements are less precise but are still encountered in outpatient settings where patients might use spoons or cups to measure their medication. Knowing that a tablespoon equals about 15 mL and a teaspoon holds about 5 mL can help technicians guide patients correctly when dispensing liquid medicines.

Dosage calculations often involve converting patient weights from pounds to kilograms since medication dosages are typically prescribed based on body weight. Remember here that 1 kilogram corresponds to approximately 2.2 pounds.

The following basic steps should be taken when performing medication conversions:

1. Clearly identify the starting unit and desired unit of measurement.
2. Determine if you need a conversion factor and what that factor is.
3. Use dimensional analysis or ratio-proportion methods for conversion accuracy.
4. Always double-check your calculations with a calculator.
5. Verify your final answer makes sense logically within the clinical context.

Consider an example: A doctor orders Tetracycline with a dosage of 6 mg/kg for a pediatric patient who weighs 44 pounds. First, convert pounds to kilograms by dividing by 2.2; the patient's weight in kilograms would be roughly 20 kg. Next, multiply the weight by the dose per kilogram; so it would be:

20 kg x 6 mg/kg = 120 mg Tetracycline needed per dose

In some cases, conversions from solid forms such as tablets or capsules to liquid forms may also be required if a patient has trouble swallowing pills or if dosing via enteral feeding tubes is needed.

Converting concentrations can also play a significant role in preparing medications in different dilutions or strengths. If concentrated solutions need to be diluted before administering, understanding how much diluent should be added based on desired final concentration is crucial.

Lastly, understanding IU (international units), which is another convention used particularly for vitamins and some drugs like insulin, ensures appropriate conversation into milligrams when needed through specific conversion factors unique for each drug or substance due to their activity profiles.

It's clear that medication conversion awareness invites an additional layer of safety into pharmacy practices. As new formulations emerge and prescriber habits vary greatly among different healthcare settings - being adept at such calculations positions pharmacy technicians as gatekeepers who guard against meditational errors while maintaining high standards in patient care delivery.

CHAPTER 5
MEDICATIONS AND DRUG CLASSES

Common Medications and Their Uses

As a pharmacy technician preparing for the PTCB exam, it is essential to have a comprehensive understanding of medications commonly prescribed in the United States. This knowledge not only aids in your exam preparation but also ensures competence in your future role within a pharmacy environment.

One class of medications widely used today includes *antihypertensives*, which manage high blood pressure. A prime example of this is *Lisinopril*, an ACE inhibitor that relaxes blood vessels and reduces blood pressure, thus helping to prevent strokes and heart attacks. Pharmacy technicians must be aware that patients often need to have their blood pressure monitored regularly while on such medication.

Another significant category is antibiotics like *Amoxicillin*. It is part of the penicillin class used to treat bacterial infections by inhibiting the growth of bacteria. As a technician, being familiar with common dosages and potential allergic reactions to antibiotics is crucial to ensure patient safety.

For patients with type 2 diabetes, *Metformin* is frequently prescribed. It's an oral antidiabetic medication that improves insulin sensitivity and decreases glucose production in the liver. Attention must be given to interactions with other drugs and potential side effects like gastrointestinal distress.

Pain management often involves prescription drugs like *Ibuprofen* or *Acetaminophen*. Ibuprofen falls under nonsteroidal anti-inflammatory drugs (NSAIDs), which relieve pain, reduce inflammation, and lower fever. Acetaminophen is often an alternative for pain relief that does not have anti-inflammatory properties but has antipyretic effects for reducing fever.

Moving on to mental health, one cannot overlook the use of antidepressants like *Sertraline* – an SSRI (Selective Serotonin Reuptake Inhibitor) that helps alleviate symptoms of depression by increasing serotonin levels in the brain. Patients may experience side effects such as insomnia or dizziness; thus, monitoring and consultation are critical.

Similarly important are statins such as *Atorvastatin* used to lower cholesterol levels and reduce the risk of heart disease. Since statins can interact with foods like grapefruit and other medications causing adverse effects, education on dietary restrictions and interaction vigilance is a key role of pharmacy technicians.

Also in cardiovascular health are Beta-blockers like *Metoprolol* which are used to treat high blood pressure and angina by slowing down the heart rate – awareness about vital sign changes is necessary when dispensing this medication.

Bronchodilators such as *Albuterol* are lifesavers for patients with asthma or COPD by relaxing muscles in the airways and increasing airflow to the lungs. Technicians should counsel patients on proper inhaler technique to maximize therapeutic benefits.

In regard to anticoagulants, *Warfarin* plays a crucial role in preventing blood clots; however, consistent monitoring through International Normalized Ratio (INR) tests is imperative due to its narrow therapeutic index and various food-drug interactions.

Lastly, medications for treating chronic conditions such as *Levothyroxine* for hypothyroidism – requiring regular thyroid function tests to adjust dosage – are often encountered in pharmacies. Pharmacy technicians should remind patients about adherence and consistency in taking such life-long medications.

Pharmacy technicians should ensure these common medications are dispensed correctly while providing critical information about their use. The importance of understanding instructions on dosage forms, routes of administration, possible side effects or adverse reactions allows techs to act as vital intermediaries between pharmacists and patients - thereby promoting safe medication practices. This overview comprises just a fraction of the knowledge base that will be tested on the PTCB exam but gives a broad understanding of various medications you will encounter daily as a pharmacy technician.

Drug Classes and Pharmacology

Pharmacology provides an understanding of the drugs used to diagnose, treat, prevent, or cure diseases. Drug classes categorize medications based on their therapeutic effects, mechanisms of action—the biochemical process through which a drug produces its effect— and chemical characteristics.

One major class of drugs is *analgesics*, which are used to alleviate pain without causing unconsciousness or an immense sensory block. These can be further divided into narcotics, such as opioids (morphine, codeine, oxycodone), and non-narcotics like nonsteroidal anti-inflammatory drugs (NSAIDs), including aspirin and ibuprofen. Opioids work by binding to specific receptors in the brain and spinal cord to reduce the perception of pain, while NSAIDs inhibit enzymes called cyclooxygenases to decrease the production of prostaglandins that signal pain and inflammation.

Another vital class is *antibiotics*, substances that kill bacteria or slow their growth. Antibiotics can be broad-spectrum, affecting a wide range of bacteria, or narrow-spectrum, targeting specific species. Mechanisms of action vary; penicillin work by disrupting bacterial cell walls while tetracyclines inhibit protein synthesis within bacterial cells.

Antihypertensives are also widely prescribed and are used to lower high blood pressure. Classes within antihypertensives include diuretics (which help eliminate excess salt and water from the body), beta-blockers (which decrease heart rate and force of contraction), ACE inhibitors (which prevent the conversion of angiotensin I to the potent vasoconstrictor angiotensin II), and calcium channel blockers (which relax blood vessels by blocking calcium entry into muscle cells).

For individuals with diabetes mellitus, *antidiabetics* are essential in managing their condition. Insulin preparations are a cornerstone for those with type 1 diabetes or advanced type 2 diabetes. Oral antidiabetics include sulfonylureas stimulating insulin release from pancreatic beta cells, metformin improving insulin sensitivity and reducing glucose production in the liver, and thiazolidinediones activating receptors that help insulin's action.

Psychotropic drugs modulate psychic function and include several categories: *antidepressants* (like selective serotonin reuptake inhibitors or SSRIs), *anxiolytics* (benzodiazepines for short-term anxiety relief), *antipsychotics* (used for schizophrenia and other severe mental disorders), *mood stabilizers* (such as lithium for bipolar disorder), and *stimulants* used in attention deficit hyperactivity disorder (ADHD).

Cardiology has its set of pharmacological agents, including statins which lower cholesterol levels by inhibiting HMG-CoA reductase—an enzyme involved in synthesizing cholesterol in the liver—and antiplatelets like aspirin which prevent platelet aggregation that can lead to thrombosis.

For respiratory conditions such as asthma or chronic obstructive pulmonary disease (COPD), *bronchodilators* like beta-2 agonists are employed to relax smooth muscles lining the airways; corticosteroids reduce inflammation; leukotriene modifiers block chemicals that cause inflammation.

Lastly, *chemotherapeutic agents* play an essential role in cancer treatment by killing or inhibiting cancer cells—it is a complex class due to its wide variety of mechanisms. Alkylating agents cross-link DNA strands preventing cell replication; antimetabolites mimic normal cell nutrients impeding cellular growth; natural products interfere with specific functions essential to cell structures division; and targeted therapies act on certain molecular targets associated with cancer.

Understanding these drug classes and their actions helps pharmacy technicians assist pharmacists in medication management and provide better service to patients concerning their treatment plans.

As we advance our exploration through these diverse classes of pharmacology in preparation for the PTCB exam, keep in mind this core principle: every medication possesses distinct properties that govern its interactions within the human body.

Generic vs. Brand Name Drugs

One of the most important considerations for both healthcare providers and patients is the distinction between generic and brand-name drugs. As future pharmacy technicians, understanding these differences is crucial in ensuring that you can assist both pharmacists and patients alike, making informed decisions regarding medication usage.

Brand-name drugs, heralded by their prominent names, are typically those which first appear on the market after a rigorous process of research and development by a pharmaceutical company. Following clinical trials and achievement of U.S. FDA approval based on their safety and efficacy, these drugs acquire patent protection. This prohibits other companies from selling the same chemical entity for a designated period—often twenty years—which allows the innovating company to recoup its substantial investment. These drugs come with an exclusive market presence under a name that is usually easier to recognize and recall compared to their generic counterparts.

In contrast, generic drugs are akin to replicas of their brand-name prototypes but are usually available at a significantly reduced cost. They come into play after the expiration of the original drug's patent protection, allowing other companies to produce and sell the same medication under its chemical name or another brand name; they do not have to endure the costly development and clinical trial phases that initially set up its predecessor. To gain FDA approval, generic drug manufacturers must demonstrate that their product performs in the same way and provides the same clinical benefit as its brand-name version—an aspect known as bioequivalence.

Despite cost-driven preferences for generics, concerns often arise regarding their efficacy, safety, and quality compared to brand-name medications. It's imperative to disseminate that generic drugs possess identical active ingredients, strength, dosage form, route of administration, and are required to follow stringent FDA regulations ensuring quality standards rivaling those set for brand names.

The inactive ingredients—or excipients—may differ between generics and brand names; these are substances included in the drug formulation that do not affect therapeutic action. Differences in taste, shelf-life, packaging, and color can manifest; however, they do not detract from a generic's clinical effectiveness. For certain medications with narrow therapeutic indices—where small variances in doses may lead to significant therapeutic failures or adverse effects—the switch between brand name and generic might necessitate additional caution and monitoring.

As cost-effective alternatives to pricier prescriptions, generics make treatment regimes more accessible while helping control spiraling healthcare expenditures. Their availability also incites competition among pharmaceutical companies to lower drug prices overall—a boon for consumer choice in treatment options.

Pharmacy technicians play an essential role in managing medication dispensing inclusive of both drug types. They're tasked with stocking pharmacies with safe substitutes when feasible, educating patients about the nature of generics versus brands when confusion arises or resistance emerges due to preconceived notions about generic efficacy.

When dealing with patients' queries concerning their prescriptions during your practice as a pharmacy technician:

1. Offer assurances about the FDA's robust approval process.
2. Enlighten patients about potential savings linked with generics.
3. Address any perceived discrepancies in drug appearance.
4. Coordinate with pharmacists to determine if certain patients would be better served by remaining on a brand name due particularly sensitive health conditions or potential adverse reactions.

Understanding generic substitution laws becomes another critical aspect of your role; these vary from state to state but generally entail allowances for pharmacists—with some exceptions—to provide a less expensive generic alternative unless explicitly contraindicated by the prescribing physician or refused by the patient.

CHAPTER 6
PRESCRIPTION INTERPRETATION

Reading and Understanding Prescriptions

Reading and comprehending prescriptions extends beyond merely recognizing drug names and dosages—it's about ensuring safety and efficacy in medication administration. A technician proficient in interpreting prescriptions can be the difference between healing and harming, making it a linchpin in the healthcare continuum.

Errors in prescription interpretation can lead to dire consequences, including adverse drug reactions, which are among the leading causes of patient morbidity and mortality. This is why prioritizing this competence needs to underline every action within the pharmacy setting. Deciphering the often cryptic handwriting of prescribers ensures patients receive accurate medications, dosages, and instructions. It's not simply translating symbols and abbreviations; it's about understanding context, drug interactions, contraindications, and patient education.

For pharmacy technicians working towards their certification, mastering prescription reading is to carry on their shoulders the responsibility of patient well-being. They must be vigilant in catching mistakes or clarifying ambiguities before they result in harmful consequences. With a clear grasp of prescription details, pharmacy techs not only ensure accurate medication dispensing but also uphold patient safety and contribute to the efficient function of the pharmacy.

1. **Prescription Basics:** When you receive a prescription, it's essential to understand its basic parts. Traditional prescriptions often follow a specific format with the prescriber's information at the top or on a preprinted form, including their name, address, and phone number. It ends with their signature at the bottom.

2. **Patient Information:** The patient's name is prominently displayed, along with their address and date of birth. This section may also include other identifiers like weight or allergy warnings. Always confirm this information with the patient to prevent errors.

3. **Date of Issue:** The date when the prescription is written is crucial because it informs how long it can be filled from that day as per state laws or drug regulations.

4. **Superscription:** The superscription consists of the symbol "Rx," which stands for "recipe" or "take thou." It denotes the start of the prescription.

5. **Inscription:** This core section indicates the medication prescribed. It includes the drug name, dosage form (e.g., tablet, capsule), strength (e.g., 20 mg), and quantity to dispense.

6. **Subscription:** Here lie the instructions for how to make up the medicine - applicable mostly when compounding is required. For most medications dispensed nowadays, this part refers to labeling instructions for pharmacists and pharmacy technicians.

7. **Sig (Signatura):** The sig contains directions for use (often in abbreviated Latin) meant for the patient – how much they should take, how often, and what method (by mouth, by injection). For example:
   - po (per os): by mouth
   - tid (ter in die): three times a day
   - q4h (quaque quatror horas): every four hours

Translating these instructions clearly for labels is vital since misinterpretations can cause serious harm.

8. **Doctor's Instruction for Pharmacy (Auxiliary Labels):** Sometimes doctors will include additional instructions such as "shake well," "refrigerate," or specific warnings like "do not operate heavy machinery." These require appropriate auxiliary labels on the medication packaging.

9. **Quantity Refills:** This section indicates how many refills are allowed. If no refills are noted or if "0" is indicated, it's a single-use prescription that needs a new prescription for further usage.

10. **Substitution Permitted:** Prescribers can specifically state if a generic substitute is not permitted by writing "DAW" (Dispense As Written) or an equivalent phrase in this area of the prescription.

Safety Measures in Reading Prescriptions

Mistakes reading prescriptions can lead to serious consequences; thus, double-checking information is non-negotiable. If handwriting is unclear, it's your duty as a pharmacy technician to clarify with the prescriber before proceeding. Additionally:

1. Know common medication names and abbreviations to spot potential errors or unusual dosages.
2. Use tall man lettering - where specific parts of drug names are capitalized - to differentiate drugs with similar spellings.
3. Familiarize yourself with dose ranges for common medications; this can alert you to potential dosing mistakes.
4. Clarify any ambiguities with pharmacists or prescribers rather than assuming interpretations.
5. Keep updated on changes in prescribing guidelines which can affect aspects like controlled substance scripts' validity periods.

SIG Codes and Abbreviations

SIG Codes and abbreviations are a kind of language used to communicate necessary instructions for medication dispensing effectively and efficiently. Mastery of SIG codes is critical because it prevents misinterpretation and errors in medication dispensing, which can lead to serious health risks for patients. For instance, misinterpreting a dosing instruction like 'qd' (every day) as 'qid' (four times a day) could result in an overdose. It also streamlines the workflow within a pharmacy by saving time and space on prescription labels, ensuring that pharmacists and technicians can work at an efficient pace without sacrificing accuracy or patient safety. In environments where every second counts, being fluent in this language is not just important, it's imperative for the delivery of responsible healthcare.

SIG, short for *"Signa,"* is derived from the Latin word for *"write."* It directs how the medication should be taken by the patient. As with many aspects of medical terminology, SIG codes can be challenging due to their variety and potential for confusion. Therefore, a thorough grasp of common abbreviations will serve as a valuable tool in your pharmacy practice.

Let us explore some of the most frequently encountered SIG codes:

- q.d. or QD (quaque die) - once a day
- b.i.d. or BID (bis in die) - twice a day
- t.i.d. or TID (ter in die) - three times a day
- q.i.d. or QID (quater in die) - four times a day
- q.h. or QH (quaque hora) - every hour
- q.x.h. or QXH (quaque x hora) - every 'x' hours

- prn (pro re nata) - as needed
- ac (ante cibum) - before meals
- pc (post cibum) - after meals
- hs (hora somni) - at bedtime

These abbreviations can also be combined to provide more specific instructions, such as "1 tab po qid pc," which would mean "Take one tablet by mouth four times daily after meals."

In addition to dosage frequency, you'll also encounter codes that instruct on medication administration routes:

- po (per os) – by mouth, orally
- sl (sublingual) – under the tongue
- IM (intramuscular) – into a muscle
- IV (intravenous) – into a vein
- topical / ung (unguentum) – onto the skin

Once you familiarize yourself with these SIG codes, the next step is understanding common abbreviations related to quantities and measurements:

- tab (tabella) – tablet
- cap (capsula) – capsule
- gtt (guttae) – drops
- ml or mL (milliliter)
- gm or g (gram)

Also integral to prescription writing are instruction qualifiers which define limits or specific conditions:

- up to – may use up to a certain amount or frequency
- with – implies that substances should be taken concurrently
- without – implies avoidance of taking substances together

Consider how these elements might appear in a bona fide prescription example:

> *Amoxicillin 500 mg capsules:*
> *"i cap po q8h x10d"*

This would translate to: Take one 500 mg capsule by mouth every eight hours for ten days.

Pharmacy technicians must accurately interpret these instructions to avoid medication errors that can lead to adverse reactions or ineffective treatment. In practice, familiarity with this shorthand enables technicians to process prescriptions quickly and helps facilitate clear communication between healthcare providers.

Remember, while efficiency is important, your primary concern should always be patient safety. This means that when in doubt about a particular abbreviation or if anything seems unclear, always consult with the pharmacist before proceeding.

Lastly, it is important to note that standardization organizations, like the Institute for Safe Medication Practices (ISMP), recommend against using certain error-prone abbreviations. These dangerous abbreviations have been linked to medication errors due to their misinterpretation and should be avoided:

Examples of error-prone abbreviations include:

- U or u (unit), which can be misread as "0" or "4," causing tenfold dosing errors.
- IU (International Unit), easily misread as IV.
- QD/QOD, where QD can be mistaken for QOD leading to overdosing or underdosing.

Handling Prescription Errors

Prescription errors can have serious consequences for patients and therefore must be handled with the utmost care and attention. Pharmacy technicians are instrument in identifying and resolving medication errors before they reach the patient.

Preventing prescription errors begins with a clear understanding of common causes. Poor handwriting, miscommunication, similar drug names, and dosage confusions are frequent culprits. To prevent these errors:

1. **Employ verification processes:** Technicians should verify the prescription at each step, cross-referencing patient information, drug details, and dosage instructions against the original prescription.
2. **Clarify uncertainties**: Always consult the pharmacist if there is any doubt about a prescription's legibility or intent.
3. **Use barcoding systems:** Where possible, implement barcoded medication system which helps match the drug's barcode to the prescription's barcode to ensure accuracy.
4. **Encourage e-prescriptions:** Promote the use of electronic prescriptions which are clearer and reduce handwriting errors.

Despite best efforts to prevent them, some prescription errors will occur. Identifying them quickly is essential:

1. **Double-check work:** Routinely double-check prescriptions filled against the original orders – especially those that are handwritten.

2. **Listen to patients:** Engage with patients when dispensing medication; they may notice discrepancies you missed.
3. **Know high-risk medications:** Be extra vigilant with medications that have narrow therapeutic windows or look-alike/sound-alike qualities.

When an error is identified, prompt and appropriate action is required:

1. **Notify the pharmacist immediately:** Pharmacists should be informed of any errors for immediate assessment.
2. **Assess the error's impact:** Evaluate if the error has reached the patient and if there is any potential harm.
3. **Inform and instruct the patient:** If an error has occurred, inform the patient sincerely while maintaining professionalism. Offer clear instructions on corrective measures.
4. **Correct the error:** Dispense the correct medication as quickly as possible once verified by a pharmacist.

After addressing immediate concerns with a prescription error, appropriate documentation and reporting must follow:

1. **Document in detail:** Record what the error was, how it occurred, who was involved, and how it was rectified.
2. **Use incident reporting systems:** Utilize formal reports to document errors internally within your organization – this aids in tracking trends and preventing future occurrences.

Learning from mistakes is crucial to improving pharmacy practice:

1. Attend regular training sessions on medication safety.
2. Review reported errors periodically to understand their root causes.
3. Engage in open discussions about near-misses as learning tools for prevention.

Handling prescription errors responsibly not only ensures patient safety but also builds trust between patients and healthcare professionals. Pharmacy technicians must remain vigilant at every stage of prescription processing – from receiving and interpreting prescriptions to dispensing medications accurately.

By following structured protocols for prevention, identification, management, documentation, reporting and continuous learning regarding prescription errors - pharmacy technicians can contribute significantly towards reducing medication errors in their practice setting.

In preparing for the PTCB exam, understand that questions may explore topics like types of medication errors, strategies for prevention, steps for managing discovered discrepancies in prescriptions, methods for reporting errors within your pharmacy team structure as well as regulatory requirements related to reporting serious medication incidents externally.

CHAPTER 7
MEDICATION SAFETY

Medication Storage and Handling

The efficacy and safety of medications can be significantly affected by how they are stored and handled. Several factors need to be considered: temperature, light, moisture, and security.

Temperature is a critical factor in the storage of medications. Most medications should be kept at room temperature, between 68°F and 77°F (20°C and 25°C). However, certain drugs need to be refrigerated or even frozen to maintain their potency. For example, insulin is one such medication that must be kept in cold storage. It's important to have thermometers in refrigerators and freezers where medications are stored and to regularly log temperatures to ensure they remain within the necessary range.

Light is another environmental factor that can affect medication stability. Some drugs are sensitive to light and must be stored in amber-colored or opaque containers to protect against photodegradation. Pharmacy technicians should be aware of which medications require protection from light and ensure proper storage conditions.

Moisture can also degrade medications, leading to reduced effectiveness or safety issues. Medications should be kept in their original containers with airtight caps until they are used. If desiccants are provided with certain medications, it's crucial always to keep them in the container with the medication. Silica gel packets often accompany these drugs as desiccants; they are not edible and should not be discarded until the medication is completely used up.

Security is paramount when handling medications. Controlled substances require stringent storage protocols due to their potential for abuse or diversion. Pharmacy technicians must ensure that these substances are stored in a securely locked safe or cabinet with limited access. Accounting for these medications involves precise inventory management practices, including regular counts and maintaining accurate records.

Handling medications also involves special consideration for contamination prevention. It's crucial to use gloves when handling medications that can be absorbed through the skin or otherwise harm the handler. Moreover, hygiene practices such as handwashing before and after handling any medication are vital in preventing cross-contamination between different drugs, especially when compounding procedures take place.

Next comes the importance of properly disposing of expired or unused medications. The pharmacy technician should follow specific protocols set forth by law and their practice site for proper disposal methods. Expired pharmaceuticals may not only have diminished potency but can also become harmful if ingested; this danger makes their prompt deletion critical.

Returning to contamination concerns, pharmacies often employ additional measures such as clean benches or laminar airflow workbenches for the preparation of sterile products. These products include items like IV bags, syringes for injections, or eye drops that require a particulate-free environment to prevent infections upon administration.

Within a retail pharmacy setting, over-the-counter (OTC) products must still adhere to similar principles of storage – staying within recommended temperature ranges and being secured appropriately based on regulations regarding theft-prone items such as pseudoephedrine containing products.

Proper inventory management plays a role in storage as well by ensuring that older stock is used before new stock – commonly referred to as "stock rotation". This task helps prevent expiration of medication on shelves and contributes towards better control over inventory levels.

Quick access reference materials like drug monographs or online databases help pharmacy technicians verify specific storage requirements on an ongoing basis.

Finally, while discussing delivery services which many pharmacies provide – special care must cater towards maintaining appropriate conditions during transport. Temperature-controlled containers may be used for insulins or biologicals which could degrade if exposed unnecessarily to extreme temperatures during delivery.

Preventing Medication Errors

Medication errors can have dire consequences. As pharmacy professionals, we must safeguard against these errors throughout the medication use process. This chapter outlines strategies to prevent medication errors, which is a core competency for the PTCB exam prep.

Errors can occur at any stage of the medication use process—from prescribing and transcribing to dispensing and administration. Understanding the types of errors and strategies to prevent them is essential for patient safety and professional accountability.

Medication errors can be classified into several types, each with its own set of causes and prevention strategies. These include:

1. **Prescribing Errors:** Incorrect drug selection, dosage calculation errors, or failing to consider patient's allergies or other medications.
2. **Transcription Errors:** Mistakes in transcribing the prescription, including wrong drug name, dosage form, or strength.
3. **Dispensing Errors:** Errors at the point of dispensing could include incorrect medication being given out, wrong quantity, or incorrect labeling.
4. **Administration Errors:** Mistakes made by healthcare providers or patients when giving the medication such as incorrect timing, technique, or administering the wrong dose.

To prevent these errors, several strategies have been developed:

1. **Double-Checking Systems:** Implement a system where another healthcare professional checks the prescription at various points in the process.
2. **Electronic Prescriptions:** Encourage prescribers to use e-prescriptions which reduce the risk of misinterpretation from illegible handwriting.
3. **Bar Code Medication Administration (BCMA):** Using barcode systems can substantially reduce administration errors by ensuring that the right patient gets the right medication at the right dose and time.
4. **Automated Dispensing Cabinets (ADCs):** Utilize ADCs to safely dispense medication while tracking inventory levels and usage patterns.
5. **Standard Operating Procedures (SOPs):** Establish clear SOPs for every step in medication handling and follow them consistently.
6. **Patient Education:** Educate patients on their medications – uses, doses, administration times, and potential side effects – empowering them to be an additional checkpoint in preventing errors.
7. **Continuous Education:** Pharmacy professionals should engage in ongoing education about new drugs, technologies, and error prevention strategies.

Pharmacy technicians are often the final checkpoint before a medication reaches a patient's hands. Hence their role in preventing errors is pivotal.

1. **Verify Information:** Always verify patient information and cross-check it against prescription orders before dispensing.
2. **Attention to Detail:** Pay careful attention to drugs with similar names or packaging that can easily be confused.
3. **Ask Questions:** Never hesitate to clarify with a pharmacist if there's uncertainty about a prescription.
4. **Report & Document Errors:** If an error has been identified, reporting it immediately allows for corrective action.

Creating a culture of safety where all team members are encouraged to report near-misses without fear of punishment encourages open communication and helps identify potential gaps in processes before they result in errors.

Preventing medication errors is an ongoing challenge that requires vigilance, continuous education, and system improvements. Leveraging technology, implementing safety protocols such as double-checking systems and ADCs along with patient engagement are key strategies that pharmacy technicians must incorporate into their practices.

For PTCB exam-takers understanding these prevention strategies not only aids in passing their certification but also provides essential tools for ensuring patient safety throughout their careers as pharmacy technicians. Remember that preventing medication errors isn't just about avoiding mistakes; it's about creating an environment where safety is prioritized above all else.

Reporting Adverse Reactions

Adverse drug reactions (ADRs), also known as side effects, can range from mild discomfort to severe, life-threatening events. They are broadly classified into two categories: predictable and unpredictable reactions.

Predictable reactions are dose-dependent, related to the drug's pharmacological action, and occur in otherwise healthy individuals. These include side effects, overdoses, and drug interactions. Unpredictable reactions are not dose-related and include drug allergies and idiosyncratic reactions. Every pharmacy technician must recognize the signs of ADRs and know the protocols for addressing and reporting them.

For the exam, technicians should be aware of several key points when dealing with reporting adverse reactions:

1. **Recognizing ADRs:** Pharmacy technicians must be vigilant in recognizing possible adverse reactions. This includes understanding both common and rare side effects of

medications, being alert to any complaints from patients that could indicate an ADR, and knowing when to refer a patient to the pharmacist or other healthcare professional.

2. **Documentation:** When a potential ADR is identified, documenting the reaction accurately and thoroughly is essential. Information should include the name of the medication(s) involved, dosage, duration of therapy, a detailed description of the reaction, any other concurrent medications or health conditions that could have contributed to the reaction, and finally, patient demographics.

3. **Reporting Mechanisms:** In the United States, ADRs are reported through the FDA's MedWatch program. The reporting can be done online or by filling out a paper form (FDA Form 3500). It's essential for technicians to familiarize themselves with this process since they may be responsible for assisting pharmacists in the reporting procedure.

4. **Communication:** Informing patients about the importance of reporting any unusual or unexpected symptoms while taking medication is also part of a pharmacy technician's responsibility. Technicians often serve as a first point of contact and must be capable of communicating effectively with patients about their medications.

5. **Follow-Up:** After an adverse reaction has been reported, there may be follow-up required; this could involve additional paperwork or providing further information to regulatory agencies or drug manufacturers.

6. **Privacy Concerns:** When documenting and reporting ADRs, confidentiality must be maintained at all times following HIPAA regulations.

Now let us delve deeper into how these points translate into action within a pharmacy setting through an illustrative example:

Example Case:

John Doe was prescribed Amoxicillin for an infection but returned to your pharmacy complaining of rash and shortness of breath—a possible adverse reaction. As a pharmacy technician:

1. First, you would notify your supervising pharmacist immediately while ensuring that Mr. Doe receives immediate medical attention if needed.
2. Next, you would document his complaints while confirming his medication regimen.
3. Once Mr. Doe's immediate needs are addressed, you assist your pharmacist in completing Form 3500 for MedWatch.
4. Information like Mr. Doe's age, gender as well as his symptoms—rash and shortness of breath—are filled out on MedWatch forms.
5. You also include details regarding his dosage—500 mg three times daily—and mention that he has been on therapy for three days.

6. It is crucial to record whether John was taking any other medications or had pre-existing conditions that could contribute to this suspected ADR.

7. After submission of this report to MedWatch by your pharmacist under your assistance, monitor Mr. Doe's status with follow-ups from healthcare providers when necessary.

In this case scenario, it highlights why it is necessary for pharmacy technicians on their PTCB exam prep path to familiarize themselves with not only recognizing potential adverse reactions but reacting appropriately both medically for patient safety as well as procedurally following protocol.

CHAPTER 8
COMPOUNDING AND DOSAGE FORMS

Types of Dosage Forms

The various dosage forms are designed to ensure optimal therapeutic effectiveness, convenience in administration, and patient adherence. Having a comprehensive knowledge of these forms allows pharmacy professionals to advise patients accurately and handle prescriptions with precision. Dosage forms refer to the physical form in which a drug is produced and dispensed. They range from solid and liquid to gaseous and are chosen based on the intended route of administration, rate of absorption, and the drug's chemical properties.

Solid dosage forms include tablets, capsules, powders, and suppositories, each with its specific use case. Liquid forms encompass solutions, syrups, suspensions, emulsions, and injectables, which can be more suitable for certain populations or conditions. Additionally, other dosage forms such as transdermal patches, inhalants, and ophthalmic preparations cater to localized or systemic effects.

1. **Tablets:** Tablets are one of the most common oral dosage forms. They are made by compressing powder into a solid form using a tablet press. Tablets can provide an accurate dose, are easy to produce on a large scale, and offer a convenient way to deliver medication. Some tablets are scored, allowing them to be easily broken for patients who require a lower dose.

2. **Capsules:** Capsules consist of medication encased in a gelatin shell. The two primary types of capsules are hard capsules and soft capsules. Hard capsules can hold powder

or granular medications, while soft capsules can contain oils or active ingredients dissolved in oil. Capsules mask unpleasant tastes and odors and can be easier to swallow than tablets.

3. **Solutions:** A solution is a liquid form where the drug is completely dissolved in a solvent. It offers rapid absorption and ease of use for patients who have difficulty swallowing solid dosage forms. Additionally, solutions allow precise dosing adjustments.

4. **Suspensions:** Suspensions are mixtures where the drug particles are dispersed throughout a liquid but not dissolved. They must be well shaken before administration to ensure even distribution of the medication within the liquid.

5. **Emulsions:** Emulsions are mixtures of two immiscible liquids where one is dispersed as droplets within the other, often enhanced with an emulsifying agent to improve stability. Emulsions can be used orally (like cod liver oil), topically (lotions), or intravenously (lipid-based drugs).

6. **Ointments:** Ointments are semi-solid preparations intended for external application to skin or mucous membranes. They contain medicaments that exert local effects or provide systemic effects after being absorbed through the skin.

7. **Creams:** Similar to ointments but possessing a water base, creams spread more easily on the skin and are absorbed more rapidly. Creams afford hydration effects that ointments do not and therefore are sometimes preferred in certain dermatological conditions.

8. **Gels:** Comprised mostly of water or alcohol and thickened with an agent like cellulose or gelatin, gels offer both topical application for skin care treatment as well as oral administration in certain cases (i.e., teething gels).

9. **Suppositories:** These solid dosage forms are inserted into rectal, vaginal, or urethral orifices where they melt at body temperature, releasing medication locally or systemically.

10. **Transdermal patches:** These patches deliver medicine directly into the bloodstream through the skin at a controlled rate over time. They offer an alternative for patients who may not tolerate oral medications well.

11. **Inhalers/Aerosols:** Inhalation therapy provides rapid delivery directly to the airways for conditions such as asthma using metered-dose inhalers (MDIs), dry powder inhalers (DPIs), or nebulizers.

Each dosage form has its own advantages and disadvantages based on factors like the route of administration, rate of absorption, patient preference and adherence factors, stability of drug compounds involved, and patient-specific factors including age and physical limitations.

Compounding Medications

Long before the advent of commercial drug manufacturing, pharmacists blended raw ingredients and prepared individualized medication formulations according to physicians' prescriptions. This act, known as compounding, is the very origin of pharmacy practice.

Although mass-produced drugs dominate today's pharmaceutical landscape, compounding has experienced a resurgence to meet specific patient needs that off-the-shelf medications cannot address.

Compounding is defined as the process of combining, mixing, or altering ingredients to create a medication tailored to the needs of an individual patient. Pharmacists may compound drugs for patients with allergies to certain additives in commercially available medicines, require unique dosages, or need a different administration form.

Compound pharmacies operate under stringent standards set by state boards of pharmacy and are overseen by organizations like the United States Pharmacopeia (USP). These entities ensure that compounded medications meet required quality benchmarks.

The spectrum of compounding is broad and includes various applications:

1. **Flavor Addition:** Particularly crucial for pediatric or veterinary medicine where taste can be a barrier to medication adherence.
2. **Strength Variation:** Customized dosages make it possible to deliver exact amounts of active ingredients suited for a patient's unique requirements.
3. **Form Alteration:** Changing pills to liquid form can benefit those with difficulties swallowing.
4. **Allergen-Free Formulations:** Excluding components such as gluten, lactose, or dyes cater to sensitive patients.
5. **Drug Shortages:** When a critical medication is in short supply or discontinued, compounding pharmacists can formulate a similar drug product ensuring continuity of care.

Compounded medications commence with a prescription where the physician details the desired strength and dosage form. A pharmacist verifies this prescription, assessing the formulation's feasibility and safety.

Two main categories exist within compounding – sterile and non-sterile:

1. Non-Sterile Compounding encompasses most traditional forms like capsules, creams, ointments, and orally ingested liquids. It is performed in an environment free from contaminants but does not require aseptic techniques.
2. Sterile Compounding involves preparations intended for use in sterile environments such as injections, eye drops, or inhalation therapies. These are conducted within specialized facilities called cleanrooms that comply with USP <797> standards for sterility and safety.

Pharmacy technicians must familiarize themselves with various equipment utilized in compounding:

1. **Balances:** Precision scales used to weigh active pharmaceutical ingredients.
2. **Mortars and Pestles:** Traditional tools essential for triturating powders.
3. **Ointment Mills:** Devices for creating smooth ointments.
4. **Capsule Machines:** Apparatus used when manual encapsulation is inadequate.
5. **Laminar Flow Hoods:** Provide a sterile work area for sterile compounding tasks according to USP <797>.

Quality control ensures that each compounded formulation meets potency, stability, purity, and uniformity criteria:

1. **Ingredients Verification:** Certificates of Analysis (CoA) are mandatory for raw materials.
2. **In-Process Checks:** Ongoing monitoring during preparation verifies accuracy.
3. **Final Checks:** Potency testing confirms the medication's strength before dispensing.
4. **Clear Documentation:** Records detail every aspect from ingredient sourcing to patient delivery to trace accountability fully.

Pharmacy technicians support pharmacists throughout the compounding process under direct supervision:

1. Gathering Materials
2. Measuring Ingredients
3. Mixing Preparations
4. Labeling Final Products

Compounding Sterile Products

Before we step into the core procedures, it's vital to understand what CSPs are. These are medications intended for administration by injection through various routes such as intravenous (IV), intramuscular (IM), subcutaneous, epidural, or intrathecal. Given their invasive route and vulnerability to microbial contamination, CSPs demand strict aseptic technique in their preparation.

To ensure patient safety and CSP integrity, compounding sterile products is governed by specific guidelines detailed in the United States Pharmacopeia (USP) Chapter <797>. This outlines the standards for compounding sterile preparations to prevent harm including infections and variations in strength or purity that can lead to treatment failures or toxicities.

Aseptic Technique and Environmental Standards

Central to CSP preparation is the aseptic technique: a method designed to maintain sterility throughout the compounding process. This involves practices ranging from hand hygiene and garbing to proper cleaning of compounding areas. For technicians sitting the PTCB exam, mastering each of these elements is crucial. The hierarchy of clean spaces—from the compounding area's general environment down to the critical area where actual preparation occurs—must be respected at all times. Air quality is maintained through positive pressure differentials and HEPA-filtered air supplied to cleanrooms where technicians work within laminar airflow workbenches (LAFWs) or biological safety cabinets (BSCs).

Equipment and Supplies

The pharmaceutical instruments and materials used for CSPs are diverse. Syringes, vials, ampoules, needles, and IV bags are fundamental supplies that pharmacy technicians must know how to manipulate efficiently. Each item serves its unique purpose: syringes for measurement and transfer of fluids; vials as containers for both diluent and powdered drug; ampoules for single-dose liquids; needles for access across systems; and IV bags as repositories for concocted solutions.

Calculations Required

Pharmacy technicians preparing CSPs must also execute precise calculations. These include dosage determinations based on individual patient needs, appropriate diluent volumes for drug solubility, infusion rates, final concentrations in compounded IV bags, as well as adjustments in dose based on specific stability data.

Compound Sterility Assurance

The maintenance of sterility during compounding cannot be overstressed. Pharmacists rely on technicians' adherence to strict policies regarding environmental monitoring—a practice that includes regularly checking air quality, surface cleanliness, and ensuring proper functioning of equipment like LAFWs.

Quality assurance processes extend beyond immediate compounding practices as well. Technicians should understand the importance of correct labeling—detailing drug name(s), concentration(s), volume(s), expiration date/time-ranging from minutes in some admixtures up to days or weeks depending on stabilization factors—and also storage requirements varying from refrigeration to freezing or simply protected from light.

Risk Levels

CSP risk levels are defined by potential for contamination which subsequently determines required environmental conditions during compounding. Low-risk conditions involve using sterile ingredients in a closed system within an ISO Class 5 environment; while medium-risk involves complex assembling or higher exposure time between sterilization steps which increases contamination risk. High-risk CSP's include making compounds with nonsterile ingredients requiring terminal sterilization.

Procedures such as sterilizing nonsterile powders with filtration or heat treatment are carried into practice under high-risk preparations; thus highlighting not just a technical skill but also a deep knowledge needed by pharmacy technicians in understanding stability issues and ensuring sterility following procedures such as autoclaving.

As pharmacy practice continues evolving with new treatments requiring compounded sterile products, so too must our skills and knowledge keep pace with these advances. The commitment displayed through careful preparation can save lives—making mastery over this intricate art not just a career requirement but an ethical mandate amid the noble callings within health care services.

CHAPTER 9
PHARMACY INVENTORY MANAGEMENT

Managing Stock and Inventory Control

The efficacy of any pharmacy lies significantly in its ability to manage stock and maintain robust inventory control. Inventory management is an ongoing process that must include consideration for both overstock and understock scenarios. Overstock can lead to increased holding costs, potential wastage of expired drugs, and reduced cash flow. Conversely, understock situations could result in lost sales opportunities, dissatisfaction among customers who rely on timely medication availability, and harm to the pharmacy's reputation.

A proficient pharmacy technician must learn to strike a perfect balance between having enough inventory on-hand to meet customer demand without over-investing in stock that sits unused. To achieve this balance, one must understand the principle of inventory turnover rate—calculated as cost of goods sold divided by average inventory. A high turnover rate generally indicates efficient inventory management, meaning that stock is being sold or used quickly without necessary excess.

One practical approach in managing stock involves adopting a computerized inventory system that allows real-time tracking of medication levels. This method reduces errors that can occur with manual counts and offers up-to-date information on which items need restocking. Pharmacy technicians should be adept at using these systems, performing physical inventory checks periodically to verify the system's accuracy.

Another significant aspect of inventory control is the proper categorization of products based on their demand patterns. Fast-moving items should be easily accessible to staff, while slow-moving or bulkier items can be stored out of the way until needed. The ABC analysis is a useful technique where 'A' items are high-priority stocks that require regular monitoring and 'C' items are low-priority ones, which are important but less critical in terms of financial impact.

Moreover, establishing good relationships with suppliers is beneficial for managing lead times—the period between ordering and receiving stock. Negotiating optimal lead times that do not interrupt service levels yet keep inventory at manageable levels is a crucial skill for any pharmacy technician.

Expanding further on controlling inventory involves understanding the concept of Just-In-Time (JIT) management which focuses on keeping stock at minimal levels by receiving products only as they are needed for sale or use. While JIT could significantly reduce holding costs, it demands precise forecasting and strong coordination with suppliers.

Seasonal demand fluctuations require additional consideration for management plans in anticipation of higher or lower than usual demand. For instance, flu vaccinations are in higher demand during certain periods of the year and thus require proactive stock adjustments.

Part of managing pharmacy inventory also encompasses handling returned medications properly—from assessing whether they can be put back into stock to disposing of those that cannot be reused according to legal guidelines and environmental considerations.

Effective management extends to controlling theft and pilferage through security measures like restricted access areas and surveillance systems. Regular audits ensure accuracy in inventory levels and deter potential theft within the pharmacy setting.

Finally, from the perspective of preparing for the PTCB exam, understanding laws and regulations pertaining to controlled substances' inventory is imperative. The Drug Enforcement Administration (DEA) mandates strict record-keeping standards that every pharmacy technician must adhere to when handling such medications.

Ordering and Receiving Medications

Successful inventory management begins with an effective medication ordering system. Pharmacies must maintain a delicate balance between having sufficient stock to fulfill prescriptions and minimizing excess inventory that can lead to financial loss through expired drugs. This process starts with forecasting demand, which includes reviewing historical use patterns, monitoring current trends, understanding seasonal fluctuations, and anticipating new market entries that may affect medication usage.

Once the demand is forecasted, the next step is to develop a reorder point (ROP). The ROP is the level of inventory on hand at which a new order should be placed. Establishing an optimal ROP requires consideration of lead time—the time it takes for an order to be delivered—and the rate of medication consumption during that period.

With the ROP defined, pharmacy technicians can utilize various methods to place orders. These methods may include automated systems where software generates orders based on set parameters or manual systems where the staff reviews inventory levels and places orders directly with suppliers. It is crucial for technicians to understand formularies, contracts, and preferred supplier lists to make cost-effective decisions while adhering to pharmacy policies.

Electronic data interchange (EDI) systems are widely used for ordering medications as they provide efficient means for submitting purchase orders, tracking deliveries, and managing invoices. These systems reduce paperwork, lower the risk of errors, and allow real-time inventory monitoring.

When medications arrive, proper procedures must be followed to ensure that what was ordered has been received correctly. The receiving process typically includes verification against purchase orders, inspection for damage or expiration dates, logging into inventory systems, and proper storage according to medication requirements.

Each delivery should be cross-referenced with the corresponding purchase order to confirm that the products received match what was ordered in type, quantity, strength, and dosage form. Products that do not match the order should be segregated and dealt with according to pharmacy protocol.

Additional steps include inspecting shipments for potential damage during transport as well as checking temperature indicators when receiving medications that require cold chain logistics. It's paramount that these products are immediately stored at appropriate temperatures to maintain their efficacy.

Every received item needs to be entered into an inventory system. This action updates stock levels and assists in tracking lot numbers for purposes such as recalls or pharmacovigilance efforts. The batch numbers and expiration dates are also recorded during this process for future reference.

Lastly, medications should be stocked according to their turnover rates—'first-in-first-out' (FIFO) method is commonly practiced which ensures older stock is used before newly received items. High-turnover medications are generally placed at more accessible locations within the pharmacy while slower-moving stock might be stored further away.

Pharmacy technicians must have a firm grasp on these inventory procedures as they play an instrumental role in managing medication supplies effectively. Strong attention to detail is necessary throughout both ordering and receiving processes to prevent errors that could have serious implications for patient health as well as the operational efficiency of the pharmacy.

Inventory Rotation and Expiration Dates

A failure to properly manage inventory rotation and expiration dates can lead to dispensing expired medications, which is not only illegal but also jeopardizes patient safety. Inventory rotation is predicated on the principle of *"First-In, First-Out"* (FIFO). This means that products that are received first should be sold or used first. This approach is vital in pharmacy practice due to the life-limited nature of pharmaceuticals. One common method to ensure FIFO is through shelf labeling and arranging products so that older stock is at the front and newer deliveries are placed behind them. This demands diligent receiving practices – checking and recording expiration dates as stock is received and then positioning items accordingly.

Stock rotation isn't just about customer safety; it also has financial implications. By rotating stock effectively, a pharmacy can reduce waste, thereby decreasing costs associated with returning or destroying out-of-date medications. Regularly rotating stock ensures that fewer items expire on the shelf, which translates to better use of resources.

Expiration dates are another key concern for pharmacy technicians. Each medication comes with an expiration date from the manufacturer, which indicates the date until which the product is expected to remain effective if stored under recommended conditions. The responsibility of pharmacy staff includes making sure that these conditions are maintained – protection from heat, light, moisture, and so on, depending on specific medication needs.

Monitoring of expiration dates can be particularly challenging in busy pharmacies, where a vast number of different medications come in and out regularly. One technique used to manage this is through periodic audits of stock. Technicians often conduct monthly checks of inventory to confirm expiration dates are not approaching. If near-expiry medications are found, they can be flagged for rapid use or returned to the distributor if possible.

It's also crucial for technicians to understand how to handle a situation when an expired medication is discovered. Standard operating procedures typically dictate that such medications should be quarantined immediately to prevent accidental dispensing. From thereon, the process may include documentation regarding how the oversight occurred and may involve inventory control systems being updated to prevent similar episodes in the future.

For high-turnover medications, expiration dates may seem like a minor issue as stock moves quickly enough that expiries are rare events. Nonetheless, vigilance remains important – high turnover should not lead to complacency about checking dates during every restock.

The management of specialty items like compounded medications or reconstituted solutions presents another wrinkle concerning expiration dating. Such items often have much shorter efficacy periods than factory-packed pharmaceuticals – sometimes only a matter of weeks or even days once prepared. Pharmacy technicians must therefore understand not only how to calculate these short-term expiration dates but also how best to label, store, and prioritize their utilization.

Technological aids such as computerized inventory management systems can be immensely helpful in tracking stock levels and expiration dates. Such systems can be programmed with alerts when products near their expiration date or when it's time to conduct an audit.

Preparing for questions on inventory rotation and understanding expiry terms will provide a solid foundation for any pharmacy technician set to take the PTCB exam. Not only do these processes play an essential role in daily operations within a pharmacy setting, but they also underscore the broader commitment professionals in this field must hold towards patient care and safety.

CHAPTER 10
MEDICATION RECONSTITUTION

Reconstituting Powdered Medications

Powdered medications often require reconstitution, or the process of adding a diluent to a powdered drug to create a liquid form of the medication. This liquid form can then be measured and administered accurately. You must first verify the prescription order against the medication's label. It is crucial to ensure that the diluent volume and type match what is specified by the manufacturer, as deviations can alter the strength and efficacy of the medication. Typical diluents include sterile water, normal saline, or sometimes a bacteriostatic agent.

Once you have confirmed the details, check the expiration date on both the powdered medication and the diluent to ensure they are safe for use. Also, examine the integrity of both containers for any signs of tampering or damage.

Next, proceed with aseptic technique—wash and dry hands thoroughly and wear sterile gloves—to maintain cleanliness throughout the process. Using alcohol swabs, wipe down the tops of both vials before piercing them with sterile needles.

To reconstitute the medication, draw up an amount of diluent equal to what's required into a syringe. Inject this into the vial containing powder through its rubber stopper. It's vital to angle the needle so that the liquid drips down onto the inner wall of the vial rather than directly onto the powder to minimize foaming or aerosolization.

Gently swirl or rotate (never shake vigorously) to mix until all powder is dissolved completely. Some medications might need time to dissolve fully; following manufacturer instructions on wait time is important here.

After reconstitution, there will be some additional volume because of adding liquid—referred to as overfill—to ensure that there's enough medication for withdrawal consistent with prescribed dosages. Never assume overfill means extra doses unless specified.

It's imperative you label reconstituted medications correctly:

1. Include drug name, concentration (after reconstitution), volume, time and date of reconstitution, expiration time/date after mixing, your initials, and storage requirements.
2. In preparing multiple doses from one vial: label each syringe with patient-specific information before putting in temporary storage.
3. For multi-dose vials that stay in use: record initial reconstitution date/time on the vial so it's known when it must be discarded (typically 14 days but varies by product).

Some additional points to remember:

1. Temperature control is essential as some medications require refrigeration while others do not.
2. Only use diluents provided by manufacturers or specified in formulary; substituting diluents can cause reactions that may impact stability or sterility.
3. Understand stability after mixing; some drugs must be used immediately while others remain stable for days or weeks if stored properly.
4. Always mix thoroughly but with care to prevent forming air bubbles which can cause inconsistencies in dosing.
5. Pharmacists often double-check calculations and processes prior to dispensing reconstituted medications; don't hesitate to consult if unsure about any step.

Finally, once prepared, always practice good housekeeping procedures—dispose of sharps safely in designated sharps containers and clean up any spills immediately using appropriate personal protective equipment (PPE).

Reconstitution is a fundamental skill that warrants robust knowledge and careful attention to detail due to its impact on medication effectiveness and patient safety. The procedures for reconstituting powdered medications are meticulous but straightforward when followed systematically as described.

Oral and Injectable Reconstitution

Many oral medications, particularly antibiotics, are provided in powder form to extend their shelf life. Before dispensing these medications, it is essential that the pharmacy technician reconstitutes the powder with a specific amount of distilled water or other appropriate diluents.

The first step is checking the manufacturer's instructions for the amount and type of diluent to be used. This information should be clearly stated on the medication's packaging or accompanying documentation. With the correct measurements, gently pour the diluent into the bottle containing the powdered medication.

After adding the diluent, tightly close the bottle and shake it vigorously to ensure that all powder is dissolved completely. Be mindful that some suspensions may need gentle shaking, while others require more vigorous agitation. The final step in oral reconstitution is labeling the bottle properly with preparation date, time, expiration date after reconstitution, storage requirements (e.g., refrigeration), and any other additional instructions.

Best practices for oral reconstitutions involve:

1. Verifying expiration dates before reconstitution.
2. Using only the diluent specified by the manufacturer.
3. Measuring diluent volumes accurately with properly calibrated equipment.
4. Maintaining aseptic techniques to avoid contamination.
5. Educating patients on how to store reconstituted medications and for how long they can use them.

Reconstitution of injectable medications involves precise preparation due to their sterility requirements and potential usage in critical care settings.

The first action is gathering all necessary supplies: vial(s) containing powdered medication, appropriate diluent, syringe(s), alcohol wipes, needle(s), and personal protective equipment (PPE). Using PPE reduces contamination risks during medication preparation.

To begin with injectable reconstitution:

1. Ascertain that you are working in a clean environment such as a laminar airflow hood or clean bench if available.
2. Wipe vials' tops with alcohol wipes and allow them to air dry before puncturing rubber stoppers with sterile needles.
3. Draw up an amount of sterile diluent equal to what is needed for reconstituting medication into a syringe.
4. Ensuring no air bubbles are left inside; slowly inject diluent into medication vial.
5. Gently swirl or invert vial according to manufacturer's instructions until all medicine is dissolved—vigorous shaking may damage some drugs or create foam.

Once dissolved completely, inspect solution for particulates or discoloration—it should be clear unless explicitly noted by manufacturer's guidelines—and draw up required dose using a separate sterile syringe if immediate injection isn't required.

Label syringe with patient's name, drug name and concentration, date/time of preparation, your initials as preparer, and expiry date/time if not immediately administered.

The best practices for injectable reconstitutions include:

1. Complying with USP <797> standards for compounding sterile preparations when applicable.
2. Never using needles more than once or cross-contaminating vials with used syringes/needles.
3. Performing dose calculations accurately prior to adding diluents to ensure correct concentration of medication.
4. Communicating clearly with pharmacists or supervising healthcare providers regarding any uncertainties about reconstitution procedures.
5. Properly disposing of sharps and other waste materials as per OSHA standards.

In both oral and injectable cases, once reconstitution occurs, shelf life decreases significantly—hence timely administration becomes critical. Failing to adhere strictly can lead not only to reduced efficacy but also serious health risks due to decreased potency or contamination.

Ensuring Proper Dosage and Mixing

When reconstituting a medication, accuracy in dosage is non-negotiable. An incorrect dose may result in subtherapeutic effects or toxicities. Various factors contribute to ensuring correct dosage, including an understanding of the prescription directions, dosing requirements based on patient age or weight, knowledge of diluents, and familiarity with different measurement techniques. Each of these components plays an integral role in safeguarding against dosing errors which could lead to adverse patient outcomes.

1. **Selecting the Appropriate Diluent:** The choice of diluent can be as crucial as the reconstituted medication itself. Diluents are typically sterile water, normal saline, or specific bacteriostatic waters, but the selection depends on the manufacturer's instructions. The wrong diluent can cause degradation of the medication or adverse reactions in patients. Therefore, pharmacy technicians must carefully review and follow the guidelines provided by medication manufacturers.
2. **Calculating Volume for Reconstitution:** Volume calculation begins with interpreting how much finished solution is required based on prescription orders. It's necessary to

deduct the volume occupied by the powder from the total volume of liquid prescribed to ascertain how much diluent should be added for reconstitution. A simple miscalculation can lead to an incorrect concentration of medicine, rendering it less effective or potentially dangerous.

3. **Techniques for Accurate Measurement:** Demonstrating proficiency in using syringes, vials, and graduated cylinders is essential for precise measurement. Syringes provide accuracy when drawing small volumes, particularly beneficial when working with pediatric prescriptions. However, when larger volumes are involved, it's often more suitable to measure using a graduated cylinder or measuring cup.

   The mixing process also requires technique; vigorous shaking can cause degradation in certain medications or create excess froth that complicates correct dosage extraction. Conversely, insufficient agitation might leave medication particles undissolved.

4. **Documentation and Labeling:** Pharmacy technicians must meticulously document each reconstituted prescription they prepare. Documentation includes batch numbers, diluents used, quantity added, expiration date once reconstituted (if not used immediately), storage requirements, and any other pertinent details.

   Labeling is another critical step that facilitates proper administration and storage by healthcare providers or patients at home. Labels should indicate ingredients, storage instructions (e.g., "Refrigerate"), expiration dates following reconstitution (not just the manufacturer's expiration date), and explicit mixing instructions if further action is needed by patients or nurses.

5. **Aseptic Technique:** Maintaining asepsis throughout reconstitution protects the sterile nature of both product and diluent. Proper hand hygiene, use of gloves where appropriate, cleaning vials with alcohol wipes prior to piercing with needles, and avoiding contamination of open ampoules are standard practices that maintain sterility during medication preparation.

6. **Quality Control:** Quality control measures help prevent errors during reconstitution processes. This includes having another pharmacy team member verify calculations and techniques before preparing high-risk medications; performing regular checks on measuring equipment; and periodic training updates on new methods or regulatory guidelines related to reconstitution practices.

Once medications have been successfully reconstituted following all protocols mentioned above, dispensing must also adhere to high standards to retain drug stability until administered—meaning correct packaging materials must be used and environmental conditions considered during transit if medications are not administered on-site.

CHAPTER 11

PHARMACY OPERATIONS AND PROCEDURES

Prescription Filling and Labeling

Prescription filling is an orchestrated sequence of selecting, counting, pouring, weighing, measuring, and sometimes mixing medication in accordance with a pharmacist's or a doctor's prescription. The critical nature of each step in this process cannot be overstated. Errors in prescription filling can lead to severe consequences for patients, making precision and attention to detail imperative skills for any pharmacy technician.

The process begins when the pharmacy technician receives a prescription from a client either physically at the pharmacy or electronically via e-prescribing systems. The first step involves verifying the legitimacy of the prescription by checking for the correct prescriber information, patient details, medication name, strength, dosage form, quantity prescribed, and directions for use.

Upon validation of the prescription's authenticity, technicians proceed to retrieve the medication from its specific storage location. If the medication is available as stock medication in bulk quantities, technicians must accurately count or measure the prescribed amount. Automated systems and counting machines are widely used to improve efficiency and diminish human error; however, manual counting is still prevalent in many pharmacies.

Additionally, compounding may be required if the medication needs individualized preparation. In this scenario, technicians must meticulously weigh and mix ingredients following precise formulations under the supervision of a pharmacist. Regardless of whether medications are pre-packaged or compounded on-site, remaining vigilant about cross-contamination issues is essential.

After preparing the prescribed amount of medication, checks must be put into place. Technicians must compare the drug against the original prescription for accuracy. It is also beneficial to consult a drug information resource to review potential drug interactions or contraindications that could impact patient care.

At this stage, it transitions us over to labeling – one might consider it as a bridge between dispensing medicine and communicating vital information to patients. Prescription labeling is a critical component that includes several pieces of mandatory information:

1. The pharmacy's name and address
2. The serial number of the prescription
3. The date of initial filling
4. The prescriber's name
5. The patient's name
6. The directions for use
7. Any cautionary statements as required by law

Attention to detail continues as key while generating labels; they should be clear and easy to read with font sizes standardized where possible—the objective: averting misunderstandings leading to misadministration of drugs.

Before finalizing any given drug dispensation, additional labels like auxiliary labels can convey supplementary warning statements like "May cause drowsiness" or "Take with food." Such precautionary advice aids in ensuring that medications are taken correctly and safely.

The last part requires revisiting our initial steps—verifying all details—at this final check stage; ensuring alignment between what has been filled and what was prescribed eliminates potential dispensement errors.

This entire prescription filling process underscores not only technical know-how but also embodies larger ethical responsibilities inherent within pharmacy practice—protecting patient confidentiality throughout every step is just as critical as medication accuracy itself.

To culminate this chapter on prescription filling and labeling let us remember it forms an intrinsic part of what defines pharmacy technicians' roles—a blend of methodical precision with unwavering attention toward patient well-being that underscores its place within PTCB exam content outlines.

Handling and Storage of Hazardous Materials

Technicians must be well-versed in the protocols that ensure safety and compliance with regulatory standards. It is important to understand what constitutes a hazardous material. According to OSHA, hazardous materials are agents that can cause harm to humans, animals, or the environment, whether it's through toxicity, flammability, corrosivity, or reactivity. In a pharmacy setting, these typically include chemotherapy drugs, biological waste, some pharmaceuticals, and various chemicals used in compounding medications.

The cornerstone of safe handling is *personal protective equipment (PPE)*. PPE for hazardous materials may include gloves, goggles, gowns, and masks or respirators. The type of PPE depends on the specific hazard involved. For instance, while handling chemotherapy drugs which are cytotoxic and can have harmful effects even at low exposures – double-gloving and the use of a gown with closed front and cuffs are recommended practices.

Additionally, there exists a concept known as the *"Right-to-Know,"* which mandates that workers have access to information about the hazardous materials they handle. Safety Data Sheets (SDS) contain this information and should be readily available for reference in pharmacies. They provide details on chemical properties, health hazards, safe handling instructions, and emergency procedures.

Another critical aspect is *proper storage*. Hazardous materials should never be stored randomly or alongside non-hazardous items. They must be segregated based on their properties; for instance, oxidizers must be kept separate from flammable chemicals to prevent reactions that could lead to fires or explosions. Furthermore, these substances need to be stored in appropriate containers with clear labeling including the substance name and hazard warnings.

Pharmacies should designate specific areas for the storage of hazardous material – typically cabinets with containment features and spill control capabilities. Temperature-controlled storage might also be necessary for certain items to maintain their stability. Locked storage is a common requirement to restrict access only to individuals who have received appropriate training.

When dispensing or compounding with hazardous materials, dedicated workspaces equipped with proper ventilation systems like fume hoods or biosafety cabinets are crucial to minimize exposure to airborne particles or vapors. Negative pressure rooms are also beneficial in containing any potentially harmful aerosols within a confined space.

Inventory management is another area where rigor is essential when dealing with hazardous materials. Pharmacies must have accurate accounting for quantities received, dispensed, wasted or returned. This tracking ensures that any diversion or discrepancy can be quickly identified and addressed.

In terms of disposal, *regulations* from agencies like EPA must be adhered to stringently due to the potential environmental impact of improper disposal practices. Pharmaceuticals classified as hazardous waste require distinctive procedures in contrast to regular pharmaceuticals or general waste materials; often involving incineration in approved facilities rather than landfill disposal.

Lastly, *emergency preparedness* cannot be overstated when it comes to hazardous materials management. Spill kits should be placed within easy reach in areas where such substances are handled. Employees should undergo regular training on emergency response protocols which include evacuation plans in case of significant spills or exposures.

The PTCB exam will assess your knowledge on these varied aspects surrounding the handling and storage of hazardous materials - from understanding what they are and recognizing associated risks to employing proper personal protective equipment and adhering strictly to regulations governing their management.

Medication Dispensing and Patient Counseling

Medication dispensing starts with receiving a valid prescription, which can be either electronic or written. A pharmacy technician must be proficient in understanding prescription orders, which include the medication name, dosage form, strength, quantity prescribed, and directions for use. It's imperative to verify patient information such as full name and date of birth to ensure the correct patient profile is accessed before medication dispensing.

Once the prescription has been reviewed for completeness and accuracy, the pharmacy technician selects the correct medication. Attention to detail is crucial here, as selecting a similarly named or packaged medication could result in a dangerous error. The technician should cross-check the product's National Drug Code (NDC) number against what is specified on the prescription to confirm it's the correct item.

Next is counting, pouring, measuring or compounding the medication as required. For most prescriptions, this means using an automated counting machine or manual techniques to count out tablets or capsules. Accuracy here cannot be overstressed because incorrect dosages can have severe ramifications for patient health.

After preparation, it's standard practice to have a pharmacist perform a final check of the prepared medicine against the original prescription. This critical step acts as an additional safeguard against errors in dispensing.

Labeling is another vital part of medication dispensing that must be accurate and complete. The label should include all legally required information such as pharmacy details, prescriber name, patient name, drug information, dosage instructions, expiration date if applicable and refill information. Pharmacy technicians should be familiar with their state's requirements regarding data on prescription labels.

The last step before handing out medication is proper packaging to ensure safety during transport and that medication remains secure until administration. Child-resistant containers should be used unless otherwise requested not to by the patient or caregiver.

Patient counseling is mandatory in many areas and plays a significant role in ensuring that patients understand how to take their medications properly to achieve optimum therapeutic outcomes. Effective patient counseling involves more than just reciting facts; it requires good communication skills and assessment of patient understanding.

Pharmacy technicians can support pharmacists in this role by initially gathering information about any allergies or other medications that the patient may be taking which could interact with their new prescription. They can also provide printed materials about medications including possible side effects, what to do if a dose is missed, when improvements may be felt if it's a new treatment regime etc.

The pharmacist will generally handle in-depth counseling sessions that involve explaining how and when to take medicines correctly, highlighting potential side effects, addressing any worries about dependency or fears over side effects and reinforcing adherence issues like taking an entire course of antibiotics even if symptoms improve before completion.

An important aspect of counseling includes discussing lifestyle considerations relevant to certain medications; for example dietary restrictions when taking MAO inhibitors or time-of-day dosage strategies that may align with circadian rhythm influences on drug effectiveness or side effects.

CHAPTER 12
PHARMACY TECHNOLOGY AND SOFTWARE

Utilizing Pharmacy Software Systems

One of the key drivers of modern pharmacy is the implementation and utilization of pharmacy software systems. These systems are specifically designed to manage a variety of pharmacy operations, from medication dispensing and inventory control to patient information management.

Let's first consider the integral role that pharmacy software systems play in medication dispensing. These systems simplify the process of translating a doctor's prescription into a patient-ready product. With features such as drug interaction checks, dose verification, and barcode scanning, pharmacists can ensure that medications are dispensed safely and correctly. The software also keeps a log of all transactions, providing a detailed audit trail for future reference and regulatory compliance.

Moreover, these advanced systems can deliver real-time alerts to pharmacists about potential medication errors or adverse drug interactions. This proactive approach to patient care ensures that pharmacists can address potential issues before they occur, thereby improving patient outcomes and reducing the likelihood of medication-related complications.

Inventory management is yet another area where pharmacy software systems shine brightly. By tracking medication stock levels in real-time, the software enables pharmacists to maintain optimal inventory levels - neither too high to incur unnecessary costs nor too low to risk running out of essential medications. Automated reordering features can save precious time by initiating purchase orders when supplies reach a predetermined threshold. Additionally, by analyzing usage patterns, pharmacies can predict future demands more accurately, thus improving efficiency.

On the administrative front, pharmacy software systems streamline billing and insurance claim processes. They interface seamlessly with various health insurance providers to verify coverage details and process claims on behalf of patients swiftly. This not only minimizes administrative workload but also accelerates the reimbursement cycle for pharmacies.

Patient information management is perhaps one of the most sensitive aspects of pharmacy operations - one that requires utmost caution and precision. Pharmacy software systems come equipped with robust security measures to protect patient data within strict compliance guidelines such as HIPAA (Health Insurance Portability and Accountability Act). These systems organize and manage substantial volumes of patient records with sophisticated encryption methods ensuring confidentiality at every level.

The benefits of utilizing these comprehensive systems extend into enhancing the overall quality of care provided to patients. Many pharmacy software packages include modules for clinical services like immunizations, health screenings, or Medication Therapy Management (MTM). They support pharmacists in expanding their role as healthcare providers by integrating these services into daily practice.

Another notable feature is the ability for software systems to facilitate better communication pathways between pharmacies and other healthcare entities such as clinics or hospitals. By enabling easy sharing of medical records and drug histories across different platforms through electronic prescribing (e-Prescribing), collaborative care becomes more streamlined ensuring continuity in treatment plans across various healthcare settings.

When preparing for the PTCB exam, understanding how this pharmacy software systems work is crucial because they play an indispensable role in daily pharmaceutical operations. Prospective technicians must be familiar with navigating these systems – from entering and processing prescriptions to managing inventory and submitting insurance claims.

One must bear in mind that while technology provides numerous benefits, it does not replace the need for knowledgeable pharmacy professionals who can discern potential issues that might not be caught by automated processes alone.

In essence, pharmacy software systems are intricate tools designed to facilitate smoother operations within modern-day pharmacies – providing a significant assist in decision-making processes while simultaneously enhancing patient care quality through increased accuracy and efficiency in pharmaceutical services delivery.

Electronic Health Records (EHR)

In the past, healthcare relied heavily upon towering stacks of paper records and cumbersome filing systems. However, with the advent of digital technology, the emergence of Electronic Health Records (EHR) has fundamentally transformed the landscape of healthcare, pharmacy practice included. EHRs are not simply digital versions of patient charts; they're comprehensive, integrated records that provide a real-time, patient-centered repository for information about a patient's health history and care.

The inception of EHR systems marked a pivotal shift from isolated care to holistic healthcare provision. These systems facilitate easy access to patient data including medical history, diagnoses, medications, treatment plans, immunization dates, allergies, radiology images, and laboratory test results. This level of access enables pharmacists and technicians to make informed decisions about a patient's medication quickly and safely.

One fundamental aspect of EHRs in pharmacies is medication management. Pharmacists utilize EHRs to review prescription orders, check for drug interactions or contraindications based on a patient's health record, and monitor compliance with the prescribed therapy plans. For technicians preparing for their PTCB exam, knowledge about EHR functions like processing prescription refills or updates to medication lists is invaluable.

EHR systems also underpin much of the collaborative work involved in healthcare delivery. Through these systems' networks, pharmacists can communicate more efficiently with prescribing doctors for clarifications or when intervention is necessary due to potential drug interactions or other concerns which could be gleaned from detailed medication histories.

Another advantage offered by electronic records is that they support the implementation of clinical decision support (CDS) tools within their frameworks. CDS tools assist pharmacy staff by providing alerts and reminders about drug interactions or other important patient-specific information that should be considered when dispensing medication.

Privacy and security are critical components of an effective EHR system as well—especially since pharmacies store sizable amounts of sensitive health information that must be protected under laws like the Health Insurance Portability and Accountability Act (HIPAA). Understanding how EHR systems safeguard this data through various encryption methods and access controls is another essential piece of knowledge for any pharmacy technician preparing for the certification exam.

However complex these systems may be on the back end—with their databases, software interfaces, and network infrastructures—EHRs on the user interface level are often designed with intuitive navigation in mind so that pharmacy staff can efficiently carry out essential tasks without software complications getting in the way.

While mistakes can still happen even with robust EHR systems in place—such as incorrect data input or misinterpretation of information—the incidents are significantly lower compared to paper-based record-keeping methods. Errors tend to be easier to address too since electronic changes can be tracked and corrected more readily.

Managing Patient Profiles

Patient profiles are detailed records of personal health information, which include but are not limited to, patient's allergies, medication history, chronic conditions, and other relevant health data. The profiles serve as a cornerstone for pharmacists and pharmacy technicians to deliver personalized medication therapy management (MTM), identify potential drug interactions, and provide patient counseling.

The first step in managing patient profiles is to establish a comprehensive record. Patients should be requested to provide pertinent information such as full name, date of birth, address, phone number, emergency contact details, insurance information, known allergies (including reactions to drugs, foods, and latex), current medication list (prescription and OTC), as well as personal medical history including past surgeries or hospitalizations. Ensuring that the data you collect is accurate cannot be overstressed. Small inaccuracies can lead to significant medical errors; thus meticulousness is required when entering data into the Pharmacy Management System (PMS).

Pharmacy technicians must be vigilant in maintaining patient confidentiality adhering to HIPAA regulations. All information within a patient profile must be considered private and treated with the utmost discretion. Access to these profiles should only be available to authorized personnel engaged in the patient's care. Proper logging off from workstations when not in use and avoiding disclosure of sensitive information are mandatory practices.

Patient profiles are not static. They require regular updating to reflect changes in medication regimens, new allergy identifications, or adjustments in a patient's health condition. Pharmacy technicians must actively seek any new information during each interaction with patients—whether processing refill requests or during MTM sessions—and update profiles promptly.

Pharmacy technicians should periodically review each patient's medication history within their profile for accuracy and current relevance. Redundancies such as duplicate therapies should be flagged for pharmacist review. Ensuring continuity and consistency across multiple pharmacies or within integrated healthcare systems is vital for maintaining an up-to-date medication history.

An integral part of managing patient profiles involves performing drug utilization reviews (DURs). This process entails an examination of a patient's prescribed drug therapy before dispensing medications. It aims at preventing adverse drug events by checking for potential drug-drug interactions (DDIs), drug-disease contraindications, incorrect dosages or durations of drug therapy as well as therapeutic duplications.

Utilizing the information from a well-maintained patient profile is key during patient education sessions. Armed with knowledge about potential side effects or interactions with OTC drugs or herbal supplements can help prevent adverse events or misuse of medications.

In our modern era, Electronic Health Records (EHR) have revolutionized how pharmacy technicians manage patient profiles. Advancements in software allow for more seamless updates across various healthcare providers making it easier than ever to keep records accurate and up-to-date. Conversely technology also brings forward challenges such as system downtimes or technological errors which one must be prepared to address appropriately by having backup procedures in place such as temporary manual documentation methods.

As pharmacy techniques and standards evolve so too must our knowledge on managing these systems efficiently for optimal patient care. Continuous education keeps pharmacy professionals adept at using new technologies and staying updated with best practices relating to privacy standards compliance laws refreshers thereby ensuring that management of patient profiles adheres to current protocols.

CHAPTER 13

PHARMACY COMMUNICATION AND ETHICS

Effective Communication with Patients

As healthcare professionals, we're tasked with not only dispensing medications but also ensuring that our patients understand their treatments and feel comfortable discussing their health concerns. Empathy is at the heart of all effective communication. When speaking with patients, it's essential to actively listen and acknowledge their feelings, fears, and frustrations regarding their health. This requires patience, an open mind, and an ability to understand things from their perspective. By doing so, you foster trust and rapport, making patients more likely to adhere to their medication regimens and seek your advice when needed.

Clarity in communication cannot be overstressed. As a pharmacy technician, you should always use language that is easy for the patient to understand. Avoid medical jargon wherever possible or take the time to explain complex terms or concepts in simpler words. Remember that patients come from diverse backgrounds with various levels of health literacy. It's imperative to ensure they have a clear understanding of medication names, purposes, dosages, and potential side effects.

When providing medication counsel, structure your information logically. Begin by discussing the medication's purpose before going into instructions on how to take it correctly. Follow this by explaining any common or significant side effects and finish by answering any questions they may have. Confirm understanding through teach-back techniques where you ask patients to repeat back the information in their own words.

Educational materials can greatly enhance patient comprehension. Visual aids like diagrams or charts can be beneficial when explaining anatomical or physiological concepts related to a medication's mechanism of action. Providing written instructions or informational leaflets allows patients to review what has been discussed once they're home and ensures they can reference important information regarding their medications at their leisure.

Active engagement is another critical aspect of effective communication with patients. Encourage them to participate in conversations about their medications and treatment plans by asking open-ended questions like "How do you feel about your new medication regimen?" or "What concerns do you have about these changes?" Active engagement doesn't end with listening – it includes directing them towards appropriate resources for further information and support if necessary.

Non-verbal cues are powerful communicators too. Positive body language such as smiling, making eye contact (while still respecting cultural differences), and maintaining an open posture conveys friendliness and approachability. Ensure that your non-verbal cues match your verbal ones; inconsistencies here can create confusion or doubt in the patient's mind.

Finally, sensitivity towards cultural differences can greatly influence how effectively you communicate with patients from various backgrounds. Be aware of cultural norms regarding personal space, eye contact, decision-making within families, attitudes towards healthcare providers, and complementary therapy usage which might differ greatly among individuals.

Ethical Considerations in Pharmacy Practice

As health care professionals, pharmacists are entrusted with the well-being of their patients. They serve as custodians of medicine, advisors on prescription care, and educators for both patients and healthcare providers. Yet this significant role comes with great responsibility, particularly regarding ethics in pharmacy practice. Reflecting on ethical considerations is essential to ensure patient safety, trust, and professional integrity.

The very foundation of pharmacy ethics is built upon the principle of nonmaleficence—first, do no harm. When dispensing medications, pharmacists must ensure they are providing the correct drug, dose, and route to the right patient at the appropriate time while considering potential interactions with other medications or health conditions. This commitment extends to staying abreast of current pharmaceutical knowledge and practices to avoid preventable errors that could harm patients.

Beneficence goes hand in hand with nonmaleficence. It refers to the pharmacist's obligation to contribute to the welfare of patients. This principle involves active participation in therapeutic decision-making that considers the patient's best interests and maximizes positive health outcomes without undue harm. Hence, pharmacists must prioritize patient well-being over any form of self-interest or external pressures from employers or pharmaceutical companies.

Confidentiality is another cornerstone of ethical practice. Patients share sensitive health information with pharmacists under the expectation that their privacy will be respected and safeguarded. Pharmacists must handle this information with the utmost care and discretion, only sharing it when necessary for the patient's treatment and within legal frameworks such as HIPAA regulations in the United States.

Pharmacists face a constant challenge for justice—the fair distribution of healthcare resources. They might grapple with scenarios where medication availability is limited or where certain policies may benefit one group over another. Ethical practice demands that pharmacists advocate for equitable access to medications and healthcare services for all patients regardless of socioeconomic status, ethnicity, gender, or other demographic factors.

Autonomy is a vital aspect of ethical consideration. Patients have the right to make informed choices about their healthcare, which places an onus on pharmacists to provide clear and objective information about medication options, potential side effects, drug interactions, and more. The support for informed consent empowers patients to take charge of their health decisions in line with their values and preferences.

During daily operations, pharmacists encounter various moral dilemmas that test their dedication to ethical standards. The pressure might come in the form of a hurried healthcare environment demanding quick dispensation over thorough consultation or from situations where a legal prescription might be suspected for drug misuse or diversion.

In response to such challenges, our professional organizations have established Codes of Ethics that serve as guiding documents for pharmacy practitioners. For example, The American Pharmacists Association Code of Ethics outlines key principles that address many of these concerns directly: a respect for the covenantal pharmacist-patient relationship; honor and dignity for colleagues; truthfulness; fairness; commitment to excellence; respect for others; a declaration that whenever personal values conflict with a professional role, we must strive towards ideals that place patient care at the forefront.

For those studying for PTCB Examinations or those practicing within pharmacy environments—it is crucial not only to understand but also to apply these ethical guidelines in every facet of practice. Real-world scenarios such as dealing with electronic prescription errors, addressing opioid addiction concerns judiciously while managing pain appropriately require careful ethical consideration.

To uphold these principles within an ever-evolving landscape—one filled with rapid technological advancement and changing regulatory climates—continuous education is paramount. Engaging in regular ethics training programs can provide critical updates on best practices while reinforcing moral resilience against potential conflicts arising within pharmacy work.

Adhering strictly to ethical standards in pharmacy practice is not just about maintaining professional reputations but fundamentally about protecting those we serve—our patients. Our decisions carry weight and consequences beyond ourselves; therefore they must always be conducted with reflection upon these principles: nonmaleficence, beneficence, confidentiality, justice, autonomy—and above all else—the health needs of our patients as our highest priority. A

Resolving Ethical Dilemmas

In the day-to-day practice of pharmacy, technicians are faced with challenging situations that require ethical decision-making. Often, these dilemmas involve conflicts between a patient's needs, legal requirements, employer policies, and the technician's personal values.

An ethical problem is characterized by having to choose between two or more actions that have moral implications that could be considered right or wrong. The complexity arises because these choices might affect various stakeholders in different ways and may align or conflict with a technician's personal beliefs.

Once an ethical dilemma is identified, it is essential to gather as much information as possible. This includes understanding the relevant laws, regulations, and professional guidelines that apply to the situation. Pharmacy technicians should also consider the potential outcomes of each option and who might be impacted by each choice—including patients, coworkers, the pharmacy itself, and others in the healthcare system.

After all pertinent information has been collected, it's time to evaluate the options using ethical principles such as autonomy, nonmaleficence, beneficence, justice, and fidelity. Autonomy involves respecting a person's freedom to make their own choices; nonmaleficence means avoiding harm; beneficence entails acting in someone's best interests; justice relates to fairness; and fidelity involves keeping promises or commitments.

To apply these principles effectively:

1. **Understand Autonomy:** Ensure patients understand their treatment options fully and can make informed decisions about their care.
2. **Practice Nonmaleficence:** Avoid causing harm by being vigilant about medication errors and ensuring privacy laws are upheld.
3. **Promote Beneficence:** Act in ways that promote patient health and well-being—such as advocating for medication affordability if it poses a barrier to treatment compliance.
4. **Uphold Justice:** Treat all patients fairly without discrimination on any grounds.
5. **Maintain Fidelity:** Keep patient information confidential and adhere to established professional standards of practice.

Once options have been evaluated based on these principles, it can be beneficial to seek input from trusted colleagues or superiors. In many cases, discussing the dilemma with someone who has more experience or who can provide an alternate perspective can lead to greater clarity on how best to proceed.

When working through these discussions and reflections, document your thought process carefully. This written record not only helps clarify your thinking but also provides a log of your decision-making process in case you need to explain your actions at a later time.

Committing to a course of action comes next. Pharmacy technicians must act within their legal scope of practice and stay aligned with their employer's policies while upholding professional ethics. The chosen action should aim toward the greatest benefit while minimizing harm.

After taking action, reflect on the outcome of your decision. Acknowledging what went well—and what could have been done better—provides valuable learning experiences for future ethical challenges. Pharmacy technicians should consider whether any changes in workplace policy or personal practice could reduce future ethical dilemmas' occurrence or difficulty.

CHAPTER 14
PTCB EXAM STRATEGIES AND PRACTICE

Test-Taking Strategies and Time Management

As the clock ticks forward and the steady hum of concentration fills the room, it is crucial for test-takers preparing for the PTCB Exam to arm themselves with strategies that go beyond mere memorization of facts. An effective approach to test-taking and time management can truly be game-changing, and understanding the structure of the PTCB Exam is key. The exam consists of multiple-choice questions that cover nine knowledge domains including pharmacology, pharmacy law regulations, and medication safety. This broad range of topics requires a systematic study plan.

A month before your exam date, create a study schedule that balances all topics. Allocate more time to areas you find challenging, but ensure you do not neglect your stronger subjects. Consistency matters; thus, aim to study a little each day rather than cramming hours into fewer sessions.

When it comes to studying, active recall and spaced repetition are two powerful techniques. Rather than simply rereading notes or textbooks, test yourself on the material. Flashcards can be an excellent tool; they force you to recall information from memory, strengthening your retention. Spaced repetition — reviewing information at increasing intervals — further ingrains knowledge.

During your study sessions, simulate the testing environment. Set a timer for each study period as if you were taking the exam. This practice builds mental stamina and helps you become accustomed to working under time constraints.

A week before the exam, shift your focus to review rather than learning new information. Create a cheat sheet with essential formulas or laws — not to bring into the exam but to solidify this information in your mind.

Now let's consider some strategies specific to test day:

Start by getting a good night's sleep before the exam; research shows that lack of sleep can negatively impact cognitive function and memory. On test day, have a balanced breakfast that includes protein for sustained energy. Avoid heavy carbs that may make you drowsy.

Once in the examination room, take a moment before starting to steady your breath and calm any nerves. Begin by quickly scanning through the test paper; this will give you an overview of question types and difficulty levels. It will also allow you to allocate time wisely.

Time management during the test is pivotal. Divide the total examination time by the number of questions to understand how long you can spend on each question ideally. If you encounter a challenging question, don't get stuck on it; instead, mark it and continue with others. Your goal is to answer all questions within your allotted time — sometimes coming back with fresh eyes can help with tougher questions.

It is important not merely to guess randomly if unsure about an answer; educated guesses are always better than shooting in the dark. Use elimination tactics by removing choices that you know are incorrect which increases your chances of choosing the right answer.

For mathematics-related questions common in PTCB exams like dosage calculations or conversions — ensure precision but also pace yourself carefully through these problems as they can be time-consuming if not well-practiced.

Lastly, most exams will leave some time after completing all questions for revision. Use this wisely by reviewing answers starting with those you were uncertain about initially.

Full-Length Practice Exams

The 100 PTCB practice exam questions below provide a sample of questions that could potentially appear on the official exam. It aims to familiarize test-takers with the kind of logic, calculation, and pharmacology questions they may encounter. Using this practice exam as a study tool can help improve your test-taking abilities and increase confidence in the material. Good luck!

40% MEDICATIONS

1. What class of drug does Lisinopril belong to?

   a) Beta-blockers
   b) ACE inhibitors
   c) Calcium channel blockers
   d) Diuretics

2. Albuterol is commonly used as a:

   a) Corticosteroid
   b) Antibiotic
   c) Bronchodilator
   d) Antifungal

3. Warfarin is an example of a:

   a) Anticoagulant
   b) Antihyperlipidemic
   c) Antiplatelet
   d) ACE inhibitor

4. Which of the following drugs is an SSRI?

   a) Sertraline
   b) Nortriptyline
   c) Amitriptyline
   d) Clonazepam

5. Furosemide is classified as a:

   a) Beta-blocker
   b) NSAID
   c) Loop diuretic
   d) Thiazide diuretic

6. Atorvastatin belongs to which drug class?

   a) Beta-blockers

b) Statins

c) ARBs

d) Calcium channel blockers

7. Metformin is used as a(n):

a) Antihypertensive

b) Biguanide

c) Sulfonylurea

d) Insulin

8. Which medication is considered a proton pump inhibitor (PPI)?

a) Esomeprazole

b) Ranitidine

c) Cimetidine

d) Famotidine

9. Clopidogrel is used as a:

a) Nitrate

b) Diuretic

c) Antiplatelet blood thinner

d) Beta-blocker

10. Which of these medications is an opioid analgesic?

a) Ibuprofen

b) Acetaminophen

c) Morphine

d) Gabapentin

11. Which of the following is a common route of administration for a patient who has difficulty swallowing pills?

a) Intravenous

b) Sublingual

c) Topical

d) Inhalation

12. The term "enteral" with regards to medication administration refers to which route?

a) Under the skin

b) Through the gastrointestinal tract

c) Into the veins

    d) Through the nasal passage

13. What dosage form is typically designed to release medication over an extended period?

    a) Solution
    b) Tablet
    c) Capsule
    d) Extended-release tablet

14. An enema is administered via which route?

    a) Rectal
    b) Vaginal
    c) Urethral
    d) Oral

15. Which formulation is intended for direct application to the skin surface?

    a) Cream
    b) Injection
    c) Tablet
    d) Syrup

16. What type of medication form is created by pharmacists through a process called compounding?

    a) Ointments
    b) Commercially produced tablets
    c) Prefilled syringes
    d) Packaged capsules

17. Insulin is commonly administered by which of the following routes?

    a) Transdermal patch
    b) Subcutaneous injection
    c) Oral tablet
    d) Intramuscular injection

18. Which dosage form can be described as a mixture of oil and water with a medication for applying on the skin?

    a) Emulsion
    b) Suspension
    c) Paste
    d) Powder

19. Eye drops are an example of which type of medication administration route?

    a) Topical
    b) Ophthalmic
    c) Buccal
    d) Intradermal

20. When administering medication via the otic route, where is the medication applied?

    a) Skin
    b) Eyes
    c) Ears
    d) Nose

21. Which of the following is a common side effect of ACE inhibitors like lisinopril?

    a) Cough
    b) Hair loss
    c) Excessive sweating
    d) Insomnia

22. Warfarin (Coumadin) has a serious interaction with which of the following foods?

    a) Bananas
    b) Chocolate
    c) Spinach
    d) White bread

23. Patients taking monoamine oxidase inhibitors (MAOIs) should avoid tyramine-containing foods because they can lead to:

    a) Constipation
    b) Hypotension
    c) Hypertensive crisis
    d) Urinary retention

24. Which antidiabetic medication can cause lactic acidosis as a rare but serious side effect?

    a) Sulfonylureas
    b) Thiazolidinediones
    c) Metformin
    d) Meglitinides

25. Which of the following medications can cause ototoxicity when used frequently or in high doses?

a) Acetaminophen
b) Lisinopril
c) Furosemide
d) Amlodipine

26. Simvastatin should not be taken concurrently with which of the following drugs due to the increased risk for myopathy?

a) Paroxetine
b) Fluconazole
c) Amlodipine
d) Gemfibrozil

27. What is a contraindication for the use of tetracycline antibiotics in children?

a) Risk of asthma exacerbations
b) Risk of permanent teeth discoloration
c) Risk of developing ADHD
d) Risk of juvenile arthritis

28. Grapefruit juice interacts with numerous medications, including statins, primarily by inhibiting:

a) Protein synthesis
b) Cytochrome P450 3A4 (CYP3A4)
c) Beta-2 adrenergic receptors
d) Renal tubular secretion

29. The use of nonsteroidal anti-inflammatory drugs (NSAIDs), like ibuprofen, is contraindicated in patients with what condition?

a) Hay fever
b) Chronic urticaria
c) Peptic ulcer disease
d) Hypothyroidism

30. Benzodiazepines, such as diazepam, are contraindicated in patients with a history of:

a) Migraine headaches
b) Glaucoma
c) Rheumatoid arthritis

d) Hyperlipidemia

31. What is the brand name for the generic drug sertraline?

    a) Zoloft
    b) Paxil
    c) Elavil
    d) Cymbalta

32. The chemical name for Lipitor is?

    a) Atorvastatin calcium
    b) Rosuvastatin calcium
    c) Pravastatin sodium
    d) Fluvastatin sodium

33. Albuterol is also known under the brand name?

    a) Spiriva
    b) Advair
    c) Ventolin
    d) Singulair

34. What is the generic name for the brand Prozac?

    a) Duloxetine
    b) Paroxetine
    c) Fluoxetine
    d) Citalopram

35. The chemical name for the drug Coumadin is?

    a) Warfarin sodium
    b) Dabigatran etexilate mesylate
    c) Rivaroxaban
    d) Apixaban

36. Which of the following is a brand name for tadalafil?

    a) Levitra
    b) Cialis
    c) Viagra
    d) Stendra

37. The generic name for Crestor is?

a) Lovastatin
b) Simvastatin
c) Rosuvastatin
d) Atorvastatin

38. Ibuprofen is marketed under which brand name?

a) Aleve
b) Motrin
c) Tylenol
d) Celebrex

39. Levothyroxine is the generic name for which brand?

a) Synthroid
b) Armour Thyroid
c) Liothyronine
d) Methimazole

40. What chemical name does the brand Plavix refer to?

a) Clopidogrel bisulfate
b) Ticagrelor
c) Eptifibatide
d) Tirofiban hydrochloride

12.5% FEDERAL REQUIREMENTS

41. Which schedule of controlled substances contains drugs that have no currently accepted medical use and a high potential for abuse?

a) Schedule I
b) Schedule II
c) Schedule III
d) Schedule IV

42. A pharmacy technician receives a prescription for a Schedule II medication. How many times may this prescription be refilled?

a) As many times as necessary within 6 months
b) Up to 5 times within 6 months
c) No refills are allowed for Schedule II medications

d) Once a month for up to one year

43. According to federal law, which of the following is required to be on a prescription for a controlled substance?

a) The prescriber's email address
b) The patient's date of birth
c) The prescriber's DEA number
d) The pharmacy's DEA number

44. Who enforces the Controlled Substances Act (CSA)?

a) Food and Drug Administration (FDA)
b) Drug Enforcement Administration (DEA)
c) Centers for Disease Control and Prevention (CDC)
d) Federal Bureau of Investigation (FBI)

45. Which of the following elements must be included on a prescription label for a controlled substance?

a) The patient's social security number.
b) The prescribing physician's schedule number.
c) Pharmacy phone number.
d) National Provider Identifier (NPI).

46. What is the maximum quantity of pseudoephedrine that an individual may purchase per month according to federal law?

a) 3.6 grams without prescription
b) 9 grams with prescription only
c) 7.5 grams without prescription
d) Unlimited with prescription

47. The Ryan Haight Online Pharmacy Consumer Protection Act requires a prescription issued by a practitioner who has conducted at least one in-person medical evaluation of the patient in which circumstance?

a) When the patient requests medication online.
b) When prescribing controlled substances over the Internet.
c) For all telehealth services.
d) Only when issuing prescriptions for Schedule I drugs.

48. Which of the following DEA forms is used to order Schedule I and II controlled substances?

    a) DEA Form 41
    b) DEA Form 106
    c) DEA Form 222
    d) DEA Form 224

49. What is the maximum number of refills allowed for a Schedule III controlled substance prescription under federal law?

    a) No refills are permitted
    b) Up to 1 refill within 6 months
    c) Up to 5 refills within 6 months
    d) Refills are permitted until the medication expires

50. According to the FDA, what must a medication order include?

    a) Patient's diagnosis
    b) Medication's lot number
    c) Generic name of the drug
    d) Prescriber's DEA number

51. When a pharmacist receives a prescription with an error, they should:

    a) Fill the prescription as dictated by professional judgment.
    b) Consult with the prescriber to get clarification.
    c) Make an educated guess on the intended prescription.
    d) Report the prescriber to the state board.

52. A prescription for a Schedule II drug can be faxed to a pharmacy:

    a) Under no circumstances.
    b) Only if it is an emergency situation.
    c) If the patient requests it for convenience.
    d) For narcotic substances intended for patients in hospice care.

53. What information is NOT required on a prescription for a controlled substance?

    a) Patient's full name and address
    b) Drug Enforcement Administration (DEA) number of the prescriber

    c) National Provider Identifier (NPI)

    d) Date of birth of the prescriber

54. Who is legally authorized to sign a DEA Form 222?

    a) Any pharmacy technician

    b) The pharmacist-in-charge only

    c) Any registered pharmacist at the pharmacy

    d) An individual with power of attorney from the registrant

55. Under FDA regulations, which of these is considered medication misbranding?

    a) Providing a generic drug when brand is prescribed without patient consent

    b) Dispensing medication without child-resistant packaging when not requested

    c) Using red-colored labeling text for cautionary statements

    d) Offering detailed drug information pamphlets with prescriptions

26.25% PATIENT SAFETY AND QUALITY ASSURANCE

56. When is the best time to report a medication error?

    a) As soon as the error is discovered.

    b) After the patient has been notified.

    c) At the end of the work shift.

    d) Once a week during staff meetings.

57. Which of the following is NOT an error prevention strategy?

    a) Using tall man lettering for look-alike/sound-alike drugs.

    b) Having a colleague double-check your work.

    c) Relying on memory for drug dosages and interactions.

    d) Implementing bar-code scanning for medication administration.

58. What should a pharmacy technician do if they notice a discrepancy in a prescription?

    a) Correct it themselves without notifying anyone.

    b) Report it to the pharmacist immediately.

    c) Ignore it if it seems minor.

    d) Wait and see if anyone else notices.

59. Who should be informed first when an adverse event occurs as a result of a medication error?

    a) The patient's insurance company.

    b) The patient or their caregiver.

c) The local news agency.

d) The pharmaceutical company that manufactured the drug.

60. Which of the following actions supports both error prevention and accurate reporting?

a) Skipping breaks to keep up with workload.

b) Maintaining clear and open communication with colleagues.

c) Keeping personal health issues private from team members.

d) Avoiding discussions about errors with other staff members.

61. Continuous Quality Improvement (CQI) programs in pharmacies help to:

a) Assign blame when errors occur.

b) Prevent future errors from happening.

c) Increase pharmacy workload and stress.

d) Reduce focus on patient counseling.

62. To effectively prevent medication errors, it is important to:

a) Work quickly to serve more patients.

b) Understand and follow all pharmacy procedures and protocols.

c) Rely heavily on automated systems without verification processes.

d) Only consult pharmacists when a major issue arises.

63. Which method is effective at reducing dispensing errors due to sound-alike drug names?

a) Increasing the volume of background music in the pharmacy.

b) Using separate shelves for storing these medications.

c) Highlighting or bolding parts of prescriber's handwriting on prescriptions.

d) Converting all oral prescriptions to written form only.

64. Involvement in which activity can reduce the likelihood of medication errors?

a) Behavioral advertising

b) Multitasking when dispensing medications

c) Continuing education specific to pharmacy practice

d) Staying logged into computers to save time

65. What is one benefit of reporting errors and adverse events transparently within a pharmacy team?

a) It prevents any legal action against the pharmacy personnel involved in the error.

b) It creates an opportunity for learning and systems improvement within the team.

c) It allows individual staff members to avoid responsibility for errors made by others.

d) It ensures that patients will not find out about the error.

66. An effective strategy for preventing look-alike packaging errors is to:

   a) Place similar-looking packages next to each other for easy comparison.
   b) Use warning labels or different colored stickers on shelf bins.
   c) Limit checking by pharmacists, assuming that packaging will be sufficient.
   d) Stock all look-alike products on lower shelves where they are harder to see.

67. Prioritizing high-alert medications by:

   a) Only dispensing them during specific times of day divulges less risk overall but creates peaks in workload.
   b) Assuming most people know which drugs are high-alert minimizes the need for additional training or attention.
   c) Creating separated, labeled areas in the medication storage rooms can minimize mixing them up with other drugs.
   d) Reducing inventory levels as much as possible ensures there are fewer drugs to manage.

68. Which document should be filled out after identifying an adverse event related to medication use?

   a) A vacation request form to take time off after reporting an adverse event.
   b) An incident report form detailing when, where, and how the event occurred.
   c) A resume, anticipating immediate termination due to involvement in an incident.
   d) A restock order form, assuming that resupply will fix any discrepancies.

69. Which high-risk medication is known by the abbreviation "MTX"?

   a) Methadone
   b) Metformin
   c) Methotrexate
   d) Metoprolol

70. What is the process called when a company voluntarily removes a potentially harmful medication from the market?

   a) Prescription abolition
   b) Medication dismissal
   c) Product recall
   d) Drug retraction

71. Which of the following medications requires careful monitoring due to its narrow therapeutic index?

a) Lisinopril
b) Acetaminophen
c) Warfarin
d) Cetirizine

72. The abbreviation "INR" is most likely to be monitored when a patient is on which high-risk medication?

a) Insulin
b) Ibuprofen
c) Isoniazid
d) Warfarin

73. A drug recall that is initiated when a medication is unlikely to cause adverse health consequences is known as:

a) Class I recall
b) Class II recall
c) Class III recall
d) Market withdrawal

74. The abbreviation "TCA" stands for tricyclic antidepressants. Which of the following TCA medications can be fatal with overdose?

a) Amitriptyline
b) Duloxetine
c) Bupropion
d) Paroxetine

75. What does the term "high alert medication" refer to?

a) Medications that are often counterfeit
b) Medications that have higher efficacy than others in their class
c) Medications that carry a higher risk of causing significant patient harm when used in error
d) Medications that are frequently prescribed by healthcare professionals

76. Concentrated electrolytes, such as potassium chloride (KCl), are considered high-risk medications because:

a) They have an increased risk of causing allergies.

b) They can cause severe harm if administered improperly.

c) They interact with a large number of other drugs.

d) They are only available in oral form.

77. A medication product has been found to contain wrong labeling information that could lead to misuse. This would result in which kind of recall?

a) Class I recall

b) Class II recall

c) Class III recall

d) Not a typical reason for a product recall

78. "Dig" is a common abbreviation for which high-risk medication?

a) Digoxin

b) Diltiazem

c) Digitoxin

d) Digoxamine

79. What feature is commonly part of High-Risk Medication Management Programs?

a) Additional patient counseling and education materials.

b) Lower copayments for patients.

c) Reduced regulation for faster access.

d) Single prescriber requirement.

80. A 'Black Box Warning' is indicative of:

a) Recall procedures for high-risk devices.

b) Highest level of safety concern without withdrawing the drug from the market.

c) Guidelines for disposing expired medications.

d) Advanced clinical trials phase for new drugs.

21.25% ORDER ENTRY AND PROCESSING

81. Which of the following is not a typical feature of medication distribution systems?

a) Unit dose distribution

b) Automated dispensing cabinets (ADC)

c) Prescription adjudication capabilities

d) The ability to send texts to patients

82. What must a pharmacy technician verify when interpreting a prescription before medication distribution?

    a) Patient's insurance information
    b) Doctor's DEA number
    c) Drug name, dosage, quantity, and directions
    d) Pharmacy stock levels

83. What is the primary goal of prescription verification in pharmacy practice?

    a) To ensure profitability
    b) To prevent medical errors
    c) To promote brand medications over generics
    d) To control inventory

84. Which technological advancement has most improved the accuracy of medication distribution in pharmacies?

    a) Fax machines
    b) Robotic dispensing systems
    c) Telephone ordering
    d) Paper prescription pads

85. What purpose does barcode scanning serve in medication distribution systems?

    a) Scanning loyalty cards for promotional discounts.
    b) Ensuring that the correct medication is dispensed to the patient.
    c) Cataloguing pharmacy stock for tax purposes.
    d) Time-stamping prescriptions for legal documentation.

86. Which system is designed to automatically re-order medications when stock reaches a certain level?

    a) Inventory management software
    b) Medication therapy management (MTM)
    c) E-prescribing software
    d) Compounding documentation software

87. For what reason might a pharmacy technician use an ADC (Automated Dispensing Cabinet)?

    a) A to secure narcotics and track their usage within a healthcare facility.
    b) B to monitor patient adherence to treatment remotely.
    c) C to enable patients to pick up their medications outside of pharmacy hours.

d) D to provide telepharmacy consultations.

88. When verifying electronic prescriptions, what element is essential for pharmacy technicians to check?

 a) The electronic signature of the prescriber.
 b) The IP address from which the prescription was sent.
 c) The date and time at which the prescription was sent.
 d) The patient's email address attached to the prescription.

89. How do medication distribution systems such as Pyxis or Omnicell help in pharmacies?

 a) They provide marketing data for pharmaceutical companies.
 b) They aid pharmacists and nurses by tracking patient-specific medications.
 c) They directly contact physicians when there's a drug interaction alert.
 d) They auto-correct any mistakes on prescriptions.

90. What is the most important factor for a pharmacy technician to consider when interpreting a handwritten prescription?

 a) Legibility of the handwriting
 b) Color of the ink used
 c) Type of paper on which it was written
 d) Size of the handwriting

91. A prescription calls for a 15% w/v solution of medication X. How much medication X (in grams) is needed to prepare 200 mL of this solution?

 a) 3 grams
 b) 30 grams
 c) 15 grams
 d) 300 grams

92. A compounded cream requires 2% of active ingredient A and the total mass of the cream is to be 50g. How many grams of active ingredient A are needed?

 a) 1 gram
 b) 2 grams
 c) 0.5 grams
 d) 1.5 grams

93. If a patient needs to take 250mg of medication Y three times a day for a week, what total quantity of medication Y must be dispensed?

 a) 3.25 grams

b) 5.25 grams

c) 4.5 grams

d) 5.75 grams

94. Pharmacy law requires that no more than 120 mg per dose and not more than a total of 360 mg/day of Drug Z can be dispensed. If a doctor prescribes Drug Z to be taken qid, what is the maximum number of milligrams per dose that can be legally dispensed?

a) 90 mg

b) 120 mg

c) 60 mg

d) 30 mg

95. You need to prepare a diluted cleaning solution at a ratio of 1:8 using the stock solution and water. If you need a total volume of two liters, how much stock solution will you use?

a) 250 mL

b) 200 mL

c) 225 mL

d) 500 mL

96. To prepare an ointment that has a concentration of medication X at 5 mg/g and you need to make a total ointment weight of 100 g, how much of medication X in milligrams will you need?

a) 500 mg

b) 50 mg

c) 100 mg

d) D)250 mg

97. A prescription calls for erythromycin suspension containing a drug concentration of 200mg/5mL and the dosing instructions are for taking "10mL bid for ten days." What quantity of suspension should the pharmacist dispense?

a) A)100 mL

b) B)150 mL

c) C)200 mL

d) D)250 mL

98. A pharmacy technician must reconstitute a dry powder with diluent to yield an antibiotic suspension at a concentration of "125mg/5mL". If the patient's dose is "250mg tid", how many milliliters will the patient take per day?

a) 10 mL

b) 15 mL

c) 30 mL
d) 45 mL

99. When compounding an IV bag with dextrose solution, if you add x grams of dextrose to produce an iso-osmotic solution, which statement below would confirm its iso-osmotic property correctly?

a) The calculated and observed osmolality should be equivalent.
b) The observed osmolality should be higher than calculated osmolality.
c) The calculated osmolality should be lower than observed osmolality.
d) No additional confirmation is required once x grams are added.

100. In compounding capsules, if each capsule requires "150mg" of Drug W and "100mg" of Drug V, how many grams in total do you need to compound "30 capsules" correctly?

a) 4.5 g
b) 5 g
c) 7 g
d) 7.5 g

ANSWER'S KEY

1. B	26. D	51. B	76. B
2. C	27. B	52. D	77. B
3. A	28. B	53. C	78. A
4. A	29. C	54. D	79. A
5. C	30. B	55. A	80. B
6. B	31. A	56. A	81. D
7. B	32. A	57. C	82. C
8. A -	33. C	58. B	83. B
9. C	34. C	59. B	84. B
10. C	35. A	60. B	85. B
11. B	36. B	61. B	86. A
12. B	37. C	62. B	87. A
13. D	38. B	63. B	88. A
14. A	39. A	64. C	89. B
15. A	40. A	65. B	90. A
16. A	41. A	66. B	91. B
17. B	42. C	67. C	92. A
18. A	43. C	68. B	93. B
19. B	44. B	69. C	94. C
20. C	45. C	70. C	95. A
21. A	46. A	71. C	96. A
22. C	47. B	72. D	97. D
23. C	48. C	73. C	98. B
24. C	49. C	74. A	99. A
25. C	50. C	75. C	100. D

Instructions for Completing Full-Length Practice Exam:

- Answer each question to the best of your ability without referring to textbooks or notes.
- Once you have answered all questions, review your responses and confirm your answers.
- Consider timing yourself while taking this practice exam to simulate the conditions of the actual PTCB exam.
- Upon completion, check your answers with the answer key provided above.

NOTE: *The actual PTCB exam also includes simulations and applied knowledge questions that cannot be replicated in this text-only format.*

Reviewing and Analyzing Practice Test Results

The journey to becoming a certified pharmacy technician is marked by numerous milestones, one of which includes excelling at the PTCB Exam. To augment your chances of success, reviewing and analyzing practice test results is as crucial as the study material itself. It is imperative to acknowledge that simply taking practice tests is not sufficient – what matters equally, if not more, is the thorough analysis after each one. Begin by examining the overall score, but do not let this be a measure of your capabilities. It's merely a starting point that indicates which areas require more attention. The objective here is not just to know your score but to understand why you've missed questions and how you can prevent similar mistakes in the real exam.

Break down your results by section and topic to pinpoint weaknesses. The PTCB exam covers several domains: Pharmacology for Technicians, Pharmacy Law and Regulations, Sterile and Non-sterile Compounding, Medication Safety, Pharmacy Quality Assurance, Medication Order Entry and Fill Process, Pharmacy Inventory Management, Pharmacy Billing and Reimbursement, and Pharmacy Information Systems Usage and Application. Identify which sections you scored less in and take note of patterns. Are you consistently performing poorly in calculations or laws? This targeted approach will allow for focused study sessions.

Within those sections that yielded lower scores, delve further into specific categories or types of questions that posed challenges. Was it multiple-choice questions that tripped you up or perhaps the matching type? Did you struggle with brand-generic conversions or with interpreting prescription labels? By classifying these issues clearly, you can tailor your review sessions accordingly.

Time management often plays a pivotal role in a candidate's performance during the exam. Reflect on how much time you take per question while practicing. If timing seems to be an issue, work on pace without sacrificing accuracy. Incorporating timed quizzes into your study routine can help acclimate you to the pressure of working within a limited timeframe.

One technique often overlooked is revisiting correctly answered questions – understand why you got them right. Is it because you knew the material well or were they correct through educated guesses? Solidifying what you know builds confidence and cements knowledge.

Moreover, mapping out missed questions against your study material can reveal gaps in content or comprehension – perhaps a particular topic was not covered comprehensively enough or was misunderstood initially.

Finally, yet importantly, make use of detailed answer explanations provided with most practice tests. Analyze explanations for both correct and incorrect answers; there are often valuable tidbits of information that could provide deeper understanding of complex concepts.

CHAPTER 15

FINAL PREPARATION AND EXAM DAY

Creating a Study Schedule

Success in the PTCB exam doesn't happen by chance; it requires a well-thought-out study schedule that maximizes your preparation time. Crafting a personalized study plan is akin to mapping out a journey, ensuring that you reach your destination of PTCB certification with confidence.

Take a moment to reflect on your learning style and life circumstances. Are you someone who thrives on early morning reviews, or do you find yourself more focused during evening studies? Do you have work, family, or other commitments that will influence the time you can dedicate each day to studying? These considerations are crucial in creating a realistic and effective study schedule.

Once you have a clear understanding of your availability and personal learning preferences, it's time to break down the PTCB exam content areas. The exam covers several domains: pharmacology, pharmacy law and regulations, medication safety, quality assurance, medication order entry and fill process, inventory management, billing and reimbursement, and information systems usage and application. Each area requires attention and should be proportionally represented in your study plan based on your level of familiarity with the topics.

As an example of diligent planning, let's create a hypothetical four-week schedule leading up to the exam:

Weeks 1-2: Focus on the most challenging content areas for you. If pharmacology is complex due to its vastness of drug names and mechanisms, allocate larger blocks of time towards it. Use these initial weeks to build a strong foundation in the areas that require more effort.

Week 3: Start integrating practice questions related to the content you have covered in Weeks 1-2. This will help solidify your knowledge and identify any gaps. Simultaneously begin reviewing pharmacy law and regulations.

Week 4: Dedicate this week to review all the content areas while continuing to answer practice questions. End the week with full-length practice exams to simulate test conditions.

Here are additional tips as you structure your daily study sessions:

1. **Be specific with your goals for each session:** instead of planning to "study pharmacology," set an objective like "review cardiovascular drugs and their side-effects."
2. **Incorporate different learning methods:** read textbooks, watch informational videos, create flashcards for memorization, or engage in discussion groups.
3. **Build in short breaks:** studying for an hour followed by a 10-minute break can help maintain focus and improve retention.
4. **Be consistent with study times:** studying at regular intervals helps establish a routine conducive to effective learning.
5. **Keep track of progress:** at the end of each day or week, evaluate what was accomplished and adjust as necessary.
6. **Make room for buffer time:** unforeseen events can happen; having spare time in your schedule allows adjustments without stress.

Always remember that quality trumps quantity—spending hours passively reading may not be as productive as an intense focused session using active recall methods like teaching back or self-quizzing.

Lastly, practice self-care throughout your preparation time. Sleep, nutrition, exercise, and relaxation are not only crucial for maintaining health but also directly impact cognitive function essential for successful exam performance.

Creating your optimal study schedule for PTCB exam prep isn't just about allocating time; it's about strategy and knowing yourself as a learner. Stick with it consistently yet flexibly, making necessary changes along the way due to performance data or life's demands, and march confidently towards achieving certification.

Last-Minute Tips and Review

As the day of your PTCB exam approaches, anxiety and nervous energy can be overwhelming. At this stage, it is critical to trust in the preparation you have dedicated prior months to. Review should be about refreshing the knowledge you've already comprehended, not about trying to cram in new or complex topics. Focus on honing your strengths rather than filling gaps that might require more time than you have left.

Let's start with a vital component of your last-minute preparations: practice tests. If you haven't already, take full-length PTCB practice exams under timed conditions. This simulates the actual test environment and can help bolster your time management skills. Additionally, it provides a reality check on areas where you might need a quick review. As you go over the results, pay particular attention to any questions you guessed on—even if you got them right. Understand why the correct answer is what it is; these could be valuable points saved during the actual exam.

Regarding content review, use mnemonic devices and charts for complex topics like pharmacology – for instance, categorize drugs by their suffixes ('-pril' for ACE inhibitors, '-olol' for beta-blockers). Such summaries are not only handy for revision but are also excellent for a last-minute recap an hour before stepping into the exam hall.

Next comes the importance of rest and self-care. It may seem advantageous to pull an all-nighter before D-day in an attempt to revise every piece of information one last time, but giving your brain and body ample rest is paramount. A well-rested mind is more efficient at recalling information and maintaining focus during the exam. Aim for at least 7-8 hours of sleep before test day.

On a related note, manage your nutrition leading up to examination day. Avoid heavy meals right before the test as this can lead to lethargy; instead, opt for light yet nutritious options that provide sustained energy release without causing drowsiness—foods rich in omega-3 fatty acids like fish or walnuts can be beneficial.

The importance of understanding exam logistics cannot be overstated. Know beforehand the location of your testing center, how long it will take to get there, and add some buffer time for unexpected delays like traffic or parking issues. Have all necessary materials prepared and packed—a valid ID, confirmation number for your appointment, a simple calculator (if allowed), and layers of clothing so you can adjust to room temperature comfortably.

Finally, nurture a positive mindset as you head into your PTCB Exam. Visualization techniques can be incredibly empowering; envision yourself successfully completing the test with confidence. Remind yourself of all the hard work you've put in—this is a culmination of all that effort.

Remember that while this exam is an important stepping stone in your pharmacy career, it is not an end-all measurement of your capabilities as a pharmacy technician. Whatever the outcome may be, there will always be additional learning opportunities post-exam.

Navigating Exam Day Successfully

Preparation begins the night before. Ensure you have a good night's sleep—the kind that leaves you refreshed and mentally sharp. Avoid caffeinated beverages in the evening and try some light reading or a relaxation technique to help you drift off. Lay out your clothes and pack your bag with all necessary items (admission ticket, photo ID, water, snacks), so there's no morning rush.

The morning of the exam starts with a nutritious breakfast. Opt for foods known to aid cognitive function like eggs, which are rich in choline, or oatmeal which releases energy slowly—keeping hunger at bay and your mind focused. Check traffic reports and plan to arrive at the testing center early; aiming for at least 30 minutes before your scheduled start time eliminates unnecessary stress.

Once at the testing center, remain calm and proceed with check-in procedures outlined in the PTCB guidelines. Don't let last-minute cramming fluster you; trust in your preparation—this is not the time to flood your brain with new information. Instead, keep hydrated and focus on mindfulness or deep-breathing exercises to stay composed.

When the time comes to enter the examination room, make sure you use the restroom beforehand; this will help minimize disruptions during the exam. Find your allocated seat and set up your workstation according to proctor instructions—usually placing any belongings in a designated area away from other test-takers.

As you begin your exam, carefully read each question twice—rushing through can cause mistakes. Manage your time by gauging how long you spend on each question; if a question is too challenging or time-consuming, flag it and move on—you can return to it later with fresh eyes.

Throughout the exam maintain positive internal dialogue; remind yourself that you are prepared and capable. If anxiety creeps in, pause momentarily for some more deep-breathing exercises—they can work wonders for regaining composure.

Remember that some questions may be intentionally convoluted or tricky: they are designed to test not only knowledge but critical thinking skills as well. Utilize process-of-elimination techniques where possible—narrowing down choices increases your chance of selecting the correct answer.

When wrapping up, review flagged questions but avoid second-guessing yourself too often; initial instincts tend to be accurate more frequently than not. Scan through other answers if time allows—ensure everything has been answered and marked per instruction.

Once completed, take one last deep breath before submitting your test. Exit as directed by a proctor—and then exhale deeply; you've done all that you can do.

Whatever the outcome of today's exam might be, remember that navigating it successfully didn't only mean getting optimum answers but also managing yourself with confidence and calmness throughout. You're taking steps towards professional development that extend beyond mere test results—they're about personal growth and being ready to tackle challenges ahead with resilience.

CONCLUSION

As we conclude our journey through the comprehensive guide to ace the PTCB Exam, it's important to remember that becoming a certified pharmacy technician not only enhances your skillset but also broadens your professional horizon. This book has equipped you with knowledge on everything from the exam structure, pharmacy laws, and regulations, to medication safety and pharmacy operations.

However, amongst all this technical know-how and strategies for exam success, the last piece of advice is perhaps the most crucial: believe in your ability to succeed. Your dedication to studying, understanding, and applying the myriad concepts required for certification is testament to your commitment to your future career.

In your final preparation phases, focus on areas you find challenging, but also ensure a well-rounded review of all chapters. Practice tests should have helped you identify these areas. Now is the time for targeted study sessions that transform weaknesses into strengths. Stay confident and manage your time wisely—nerves can be as significant an obstacle as any knowledge gap on the day of the exam.

Navigating the world of pharmacy is an ongoing learning experience even after passing the PTCB Exam. Keep up-to-date with new laws, drugs, and technology changes that continuously shape the healthcare landscape. Embrace this calling with professionalism and ethical integrity; remember that at the core of your work are patients whose lives you can impact positively through expertise and compassion.

Go into your exam equipped not just with facts but with the assurance that you are ready. Good luck on your PTCB Exam and in your future career as a certified pharmacy technician.